SALVESTROLS
Nature's defence against cancer:
Linking diet and cancer

Brian A Schaefer

Wishing you all the best Hans

Brian

Salvestrol® is a registered trademark of Salvestrol Natural Products Ltd.

Library and Archives Canada Cataloguing in Publication

Salvestrols : nature's defence against cancer.

Includes bibliographical references and index.
ISBN 978-0-9783274-0-8

1. Phytochemicals--Health aspects. 2. Cancer--Prevention. 3. Cancer--Diet therapy. 4. Resveratrol--Health aspects. 5. Fruit--Therapeutic use. 6. Vegetables--Therapeutic use. I. Title.

RC262.S37 2007   616.99'40654   C2007-901942-0

The front cover photo – © candysp - Fotolia.com
Book Design – SpicaBookDesign (www.spicabookdesign.com)

Published in Canada.

*Dedicated to the next generation
who provide a continual source of inspiration and entertain-
ment. May cancer be to them nothing more than
the common cold has been to our generation.*

DISCLAIMER

The intent of this book is to provide a general introduction to salvestrols and the individuals that discovered them. Salvestrols are a relatively recent nutritional discovery. The science underlying salvestrols is advancing at such a pace that any effort at providing a definitive source of information on salvestrols will be out of step with the most recent advances by the time it is published.

This book is not intended as a medical or nutritional reference. Neither is it intended as a definitive source of information about salvestrols. People requiring expert assistance in medical or nutritional matters should consult a professional. This book should not be used in the diagnosis of any medical condition.

Every effort has been made to provide complete, accurate and timely information. However, there may be mistakes both typographical and in content. The reader is well advised to use this book as a general guide from which they can conduct their own research.

The author and copyright holder shall have neither liability nor responsibility to any entity or person with respect to any loss or damage caused, or alleged to be caused, directly or indirectly by the concepts or information contained in this book.

PREFACE

I should get the confessions out of the way right away. I am not a medical doctor. My promising career in medicine came to an abrupt end at the age of five when I got busted for practising medicine without a license in my parent's garage. In my defence the patient was enjoying exceptional health under my care but at the time no one was in a mood to listen to reason.

Actually I work in the software industry, specifically with artificial intelligence software for laboratory medicine – software that assists doctors in complying with best practice guidelines and the expertise of clinical pathologists when ordering and interpreting laboratory tests for their patients. Software that brings the specialist knowledge of pathology from the laboratory to the point of care. This work takes me to England on a very regular basis as it is the European health departments that are interested in the economic and medical efficiencies of such systems. This line of work also necessitates that I spend a good deal of time reading medical literature and news in general and British medical literature and news in particular.

While in England in July of 2001 I came across a news article that I found particularly intriguing: BBC News Health, Friday, 27 July, 2001, 17:09 GMT 18:09 UK, *Cancer drug raises hopes of cure,* http://news.bbc.co.uk/1/hi/health/1460757.stm My father had just died of cancer a few months earlier so I was still quite oriented to anything that indicated hope for people suffering from cancer.

The article highlighted the work of an English medicinal chemist, Professor Gerry Potter. The work represented a significant departure from the majority of papers that I had read in the area of cancer research so I looked for further references to his work. This of course led me to the work of his close colleague Professor Dan Burke. I found the work of these two men fascinating and inspiring a much greater sense of hope for the future of cancer sufferers than anything that I had come across before.

I made a point of contacting Professor Potter to learn more about this work. Through this initial contact I have had the good fortune of meeting Professor Dan Burke, Anthony Daniels and many other members of this team. Through the friendships that have followed I have had the opportunity to stay in close contact with their exceptionally fast paced research activities.

This research has led to a molecular level explanation of the link between diet and cancer with obvious implications for those suffering from cancer or at risk. The work of this team, however, is not well known outside of England and English academia in particular. This book is an attempt to bring this work to the public in a succinct and readable fashion. Hopefully, I will be able to impart some of my enthusiasm for this work to the reader and more importantly some of the knowledge that gives rise to my enthusiasm.

ACKNOWLEDGEMENTS

Many thanks to Lorna Hancock of the Health Action Network Society for the photographs of Prof. Gerry Potter, Prof. Dan Burke and Anthony Daniels.

Thanks also to Doug Robb for the 'Monastery Story'.

Thanks are also due to Gerry Potter, Dan Burke, Anthony Daniels and the Health Action Network Society for bringing this research to the Canadian public through their lecture series and DVDs.

Many thanks to Iraida Garcia and Mikel Iturrioz for their translation of this book into Spanish. Iraida is now fluent in Spanish, English and Canadian!

I wish to thank Isabelle Eini, Kathy Thammavong, Ian Morrison, Cassandra Miller, Mike Wakeman, Katolen Yardley, Graham Boyes, Catherine Dooner, Frances Fuller, Luke Daniels, Helen Bailey, Robbie Wood, Darragh Hammond, Dominic Galvin, David Vousden, Tommy & Irene Kobberskov, Kevin Coyne, Jim Stott and Mikel Iturrioz for their valuable comments on the various drafts of this book.

Many thanks to Gerry Potter for his kind permission to reproduce the 'Green and Red Diet' along with Figures 1 and 2 here. Thanks to Dan Burke for his kind permission to reproduce the silent growth of cancer figure (Figure 3) and many thanks to Anthony Daniels of Nature's Defence for his kind permission to reproduce some of the 'Salvestrol Rich Recipes' here.

Great thanks to Bev, Meg and Sam for your sustaining level of support, encouragement and input through all my endeavours.

Eat your vegetables.

❖MOM (VARIOUS DATES)

TABLE OF CONTENTS

1.
INTRODUCTION

Cancer is the biggest failure of twentieth century medicine ... and the conventional treatments that are available will continue to be. But the new molecular biology, the human genome project, has revolutionised everything. The key to it are targets – molecules that are present in cancer cells and virtually absent or completely absent in normal cells. Once you have such a target or tumour marker you can devise treatments.

❖ DAN BURKE, PH.D.

Books about cancer usually start off with statements and statistics about the prevalence of the disease and the particular incidence rates of the most common cancers. Five-year survival rates and discussion of the billions of dollars that pour into cancer research from all of the charity sponsored 'Run for a Cure' events are also often reported.

At this time we no longer need to read about such things. Cancer is now part of our daily experience. We see the cancer charity advertisements on prime time television and most of our cities host beautiful, new, architect designed buildings devoted to cancer. In the developed world I suspect that there is no adult that has not witnessed a relative, close friend or acquaintance, suffer or die from cancer. Most people, young or old, would have been through this experience numerous times. Consequently, we know how long our friends and relatives live once diagnosed with cancer.

While chatting with friends at the children's school field, football pitch, equestrian ring or boxing gym, raise the topic of cancer and the stories will follow:

"One of the mothers in our neighbourhood was not feeling well a while ago. She went to the doctor and after a few tests was diagnosed with cancer. She died in the midst of the chemotherapy and radiotherapy three weeks after she was diagnosed! She was only forty-three!"

"A good friend of mine just died of cancer too. He went through the chemotherapy and a huge operation for kidney cancer and was told that everything looked good. To celebrate he and his wife got pregnant with their second child. When he visited the head of renal oncology he mentioned that the surgeon said that he had got everything out and wondered why he needed this appointment. She just laughed and said 'you will be back in here within a year with bone cancer and that's what is going to kill you.' He died of bone cancer before their second child was born! He always referred to the head of renal oncology as 'Dr. Death' after that comment."

"That reminds me of my friend. She was diagnosed with lymphoma. She went through a huge amount of chemotherapy, full radiation treatment and a bone marrow transplant. She was told that everything looked good. Her family had a big celebration. About a week after the celebration she was diagnosed with multiple digestive tract tumours and died within a few months."

"My father died of cancer. He was admitted to a gerontology ward because they thought that he needed some rehab to increase his mobility. When he didn't respond to the rehab they discovered that he had cancer in his lung and his back. They did radiotherapy on the tumour in his vertebrae but didn't tell him in advance that the tumour would initially swell before it potentially shrunk. As the tumour swelled from the radiation the pain from the vertebrae cracking was so intense that massive amounts of morphine were given to him. He was dead within a couple of weeks of that."

[These stories were told to the author by friends and family. They have been fictionalised here for readability and to protect privacy.]

We don't need to hear about women getting breast cancer, men getting prostate cancer or citizens getting digestive tract cancers because we know them. We have been to their hospital beds and to their funerals. We have been to the hospital beds and the funerals of those with brain tumours, leukaemia, ovarian cancer and every other type of cancer. Their stories form part of our conversation while we watch our children play football, hockey or whatever else they may be involved with. Their stories leave us with the impression that if the cancer agencies took over air travel few would reach their destination and the food would be worse!

During one such conversation I heard a very different cancer story. The fellow that I was talking to was always good for different stories and this one was certainly true to form. Some people just have those lives that give rise to good but different stories:

"Many years ago, before we all had children, a couple of buddies and I headed off to the Orient looking for fun, women and adventure. One of my buddies took to the Orient in a big way, stayed behind and found a job in Hong Kong. In Hong Kong he continued to pursue fun, women and adventure long after my other buddy and I had returned home, married and started our families. He had the life that many young men envy. He made good money, had many girlfriends, was well known to many bartenders and waiters in a broad array of establishments and enjoyed plenty of travel. Make money and enjoy that money was his philosophy and I always found it reassuring that someone was out there enjoying that kind of life.

At a certain point my buddy didn't feel well and knew that it wasn't just a hangover. Went to the doctor and after some extensive testing was told that he had advanced, terminal cancer and he should get his affairs in order – different sorts of affairs than he was used to!

With this news my buddy thought to himself 'oh crap, I'm dying and I haven't even reached an age to start thinking about things like dying, my legacy or spirituality. I need to get away from things and find a place to think about this.' [If they ever do a movie about this man's life I think Hugh Grant would be ideal in the lead role!].

Now given my buddy's lifestyle he made an uncharacteristic choice. He knew that the East was full of monasteries and figured that they had to be peaceful places where a guy could collect his thoughts, so off he went in search of a monastery. He found one, told them his situation and asked if he could stay a while so that he could reflect on his situation and life in general.

The monks took him in but insisted that he had to eat exactly what they gave him. The monks provided him with a diet that was almost exclusively fruits and fruit juices, provided daily, in great abundance. A year and a half later he left the monastery completely free of cancer!"

You have to admit that this is a better cancer story than the previous ones! An optimistic cancer story – now that's refreshing!

You are probably thinking 'how could this be? How could this diet bring about such a marked change in this fellow's health? How could these Monks know what to give him?'

In the chapters that follow I will describe the discoveries of two English cancer researchers, a pharmacologist and a medicinal chemist, that make sense out of the monastery cancer story. I will describe each of the discoveries in their own right and then show how they come together to form a nutritional theory of cancer prevention and treatment that is available to all of us. This theory provides a mechanism to explain the link between diet and cancer. This is done in the belief that as more people know about these discoveries we will start to enjoy more stories, in our various conversations, like the monastery story and fewer like those that we are used to.

By the end of this book I hope that you will have a good understanding of how the monks did exactly the right thing for this man and a good understanding of the science that explains how their diet could treat his cancer. With this understanding you will be better able to make certain health related, dietary changes without having to go to the monastery!

To begin I will introduce the two main scientists: Professor Gerry Potter and Professor Dan Burke.

PROFESSOR GERRY POTTER

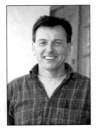

Gerry Potter is a professor of medicinal chemistry in the School of Pharmacy at De Montfort University in Leicester, England. In this department he is Director of the Cancer Drug Discovery Group, a group dedicated to the development and discovery of tumour selective agents for the safe treatment of cancer.

Professor Potter had his first experience with cancer at the age of four. His aunt died of cancer and this experience had a profound influence on his subsequent career.

He studied chemistry as an undergraduate and completed a final year project on anticancer agents. This took him to the University of Manchester where he investigated cytochrome P450 enzymes. A Ph.D. in Medicinal Chemistry was subsequently obtained from the University of London's Institute of Cancer Research. During his final year of doctoral studies Professor Potter was awarded the SmithKlineBeecham Prize for Chirality in Drug Design and Synthesis.

With his Ph.D., in hand Dr. Potter designed and synthesised selective drugs for breast and prostate cancer at the Institute of Cancer Research. His prostate cancer drug, Abiraterone acetate, has recently been licensed as a last line treatment for prostate cancer (at this point it is exceptionally difficult to get a drug licensed as a first line treatment regardless of the drugs performance). This drug is actually an enzyme inhibitor rather than chemotherapy per se. CYP 17 is a human enzyme involved in androgen and oestrogen biosynthesis. Abiraterone inhibits this enzyme shutting off this biosynthesis. Abiraterone is currently working its way through the remaining clinical trial process and the results so far have been exceptional *(Attart, et al., 2009)*.

This work subsequently took him to Cambridge where he continued developing chiral (compounds having different left and right-handed forms) anticancer agents. While at Cambridge he was awarded the Royal Society of Chemistry Award for Industrial Innovation. Within a year of receiving this award he was offered his Professorship at De Montfort University. Professor Potter has recently won his third Royal Society of Chemistry Award for Industrial Innovation for his design and development of Abiraterone acetate. He is the only scientist to win this award more than once *(Schaefer, B., 2012)*.

This cumulative experience pointed to a number of shortcomings of existing anti-cancer agents and helped to form a central theme of his research. Conventional anti-cancer agents are generally toxic, that is, they lack selectivity. As Stellman and Zoloth point out in their literature review of cancer chemotherapeutic agents as occupational hazards, "There is no speculation, however, about the toxicity of most of the cancer chemotherapeutic agents" *(Stellman, JM; Zoloth, SR, 1986)*. Most are equally toxic to healthy tissue as they are to cancerous tissue (e.g., Methotrexate) *(Potter, G., 2005)*. Some are more toxic to healthy tissue than cancerous tissue (e.g., Taxol, Doxorubicin, 5-Fluorouracil) *(Potter, G., 2005)*. Still others are carcinogenic tumour promoters (e.g., Chlorambucil, Melphalan) while others are both carcinogenic and mutagenic, a situation that can lead to induction of highly aggressive secondary cancers *(Potter,*

G., 2005). Indeed, investigations into the health risks of occupational exposure to anticancer (antineoplastic) drugs have pointed to the increased risk of cancer among health care professionals exposed to these drugs as well as an increased incidence of spontaneous abortions and malformation of the offspring of oncology nurses (*Sorsa, et al., 1985; Skov, et al., 1990: Skov, et al., 1992*).

Professor Potter is author of over 60 research publications. This research has resulted in his successful patenting of 20 anticancer agents. A common theme throughout his research is the quest for anticancer agents that are selective and harmless to healthy tissue. This research has recently taken Professor Potter into a search for natural anticancer agents that are selective, effective and without side effects. It is this recent research that forms the foundation of the Salvestrol Concept, the focus of this book.

PROFESSOR DAN BURKE

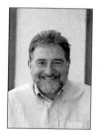

Dan Burke is Emeritus Professor of Pharmaceutical Metabolism after recently stepping down as Dean of Science at Sunderland University. He is currently the Head of Research at Nature's Defence (UK) Ltd., in Syston, Leicester, England.

Professor Burke has devoted his career to cancer. The causes of cancer, its detection, prevention and treatment have all been major components of his research.

He studied biochemistry as an undergraduate and received a First Class Honours degree from the University of London. This earned him a place in the Ph.D. program at the University of Surrey where he conducted research on drug metabolism.

During the 1970's Professor Burke invented a set of biochemical tests known as the EROD (ethoxyresorufin-*O*-deethylase) assays. These assays are the premier method of quantifying the activity of CYP enzymes and Prof. Burke is the father of this entire line of work. The EROD assays are fundamental research tools used world-wide in industry and academia alike to facilitate scientific investigations.

Professor Burke served on faculty of the Aberdeen University medical school for nearly twenty years. It is here that he was offered his professorship and became recognised as an expert on the metabolism, toxicity and interactions of drugs and environmental chemicals. In particular he specialised in the cytochrome P450 enzyme system. His research group discovered that the CYP1B1 enzyme was intrinsic to cancer cells but absent from healthy tissue. This discovery has stimulated new research on cancer detection, development of new drugs and anticancer vaccines world-wide.

From Aberdeen he became Head of the School of Pharmacy at De Montfort University. At De Montfort University Professor Burke extended his expertise to include the metabolism, toxicity and interactions of natural compounds. In particular the role that cytochrome P450 enzymes play in these processes.

Professor Burke is author of over 200 research publications that span an academic career of thirty-five years. Professor Burke's pioneering work with the CYP1B1 enzyme enabled the development of the Salvestrol Concept.

2.

DISCOVERY OF
A UNIVERSAL CANCER
MARKER

People who say it cannot be done should not
interrupt those who are doing it.

❖ GEORGE BERNARD SHAW

Development of new cancer treatments and discovery of
new cancer markers are far too often cancer specific. We
have all come across the announcements of new treatments for breast cancer, prostate cancer and the like.
Teams of researchers are devoted to single cancers and
as more and more money pours in, research centres are
opening that are devoted to research focused on specific
cancers.

Against this backdrop the "Holy Grail" of cancer research remains twofold. To discover a single target for ther-

apeutic intervention that would work across the enormous array of cancers, regardless of their oncogenic origins, and across all stages of cancer from dysplastic to metastatic. Secondly, to discover a single marker to detect and track the cancer's progress or decline. To date the discovery of this "Holy Grail" of cancer has been as elusive as finding the Holy Grail of biblical fame.

Cytochrome P450 enzymes, otherwise known as CYP enzymes (pronounced 'sip' enzymes) have become the subject of increasing research activity over the past decade. At present 57 P450 genes and 29 pseudogenes have been identified in humans (*McFadyen MCE, et al., 2004*). Many more exist in other organisms.

Cytochrome P450 enzymes constitute a host of enzymes that occur throughout nature. There are presently around 3,800 of these enzymes that have been identified. They occur in humans, mammals, fish, plants, fungi, bacteria, etc. Of greatest interest to cancer researchers are the 57 cytochrome P450 enzymes that exist in humans.

These enzymes utilise iron, at their core, to oxidise various compounds that enter the body. Given this they are sometimes referred to as hemeproteins. It is the oxidisation or hydroxylation action that enables these enzymes to make many drugs and toxins water-soluble. Over the expanse of human history it has been these CYP enzymes that enabled our forefathers to clear natural toxins from their bodies. Today this water solubility, predominantly, enables us to clear drugs and chemical toxins from the body. It is this drug and toxin metabolism by CYP enzymes that has attracted the attention of researchers worldwide. Indeed, without the CYP enzymes we would likely overdose on pharmaceuticals and toxins alike.

One particular CYP enzyme has another property,

quite distinct from drug and toxin metabolism - a property that has enormous implications for cancer research. The CYP1B1 enzyme (pronounced 'sip one be one') is distinguished from the other CYP enzymes by its presence in cancer cells and its absence in healthy tissue.

Just over a decade ago a team of researchers in the Department of Pathology, University of Aberdeen, Scotland, under the direction of Professor Dan Burke, reported that CYP1B1 was present in soft tissue sarcomas *(Murray GI., et al., 1993)* while being absent from healthy tissue. This was certainly an interesting result, but it took a few more years of further research by this team to really catch the interest of the international research community and convince them of the importance of CYP1B1.

In 1995 this team reported that CYP1B1 was found in breast cancer tumours *(McKay J., et al. 1995)*. By 1997, Professor Burke's team reported that CYP1B1 was present in a broad array of tumours including cancers of the breast, colon, lung, oesophagus, skin, lymph node, brain, and testis with no detectable presence in healthy tissue *(Murray GI., et al., 1997)*. Given this prevalence researchers have been continuing to test cancer cells for the presence of CYP1B1. CYP1B1 is expressed in all of the cancers tested to date and distinguishes itself through its pervasiveness in cancer cells and its absence in healthy tissue.

These research results combine to indicate that CYP1B1 could be both a universal cancer target for therapeutic intervention as well as a universal marker for the detection of cancer and the monitoring of cancer progress or decline. As incredible a find as this is, there is more to the CYP1B1 discovery.

Not only is CYP1B1 present across all types of cancer tested to date, it is also found throughout all stages of cancer from precancerous dysplastic cells, throughout primary cancer cells and the metastases of those cancer cells (*McFadyen MCE., et al., 2001, Gibson, P. et al., 2003*). This makes CYP1B1 a truly intrinsic property of cancer cells. (See Appendix 1 for a partial list of cancers cited in the scientific literature that express CYP1B1).

This property of CYP1B1 represents a realisation of the "Holy Grail" of cancer research. CYP1B1 provides the foundation for broad-based therapeutic intervention from cancer prevention, through to the treatment of advanced stage, metastatic disease as well as the monitoring of cancer progress and decline.

IMMUNOHISTOCHEMICAL STAINING FOR CYP1B1

The way in which researchers screen cells for the presence of CYP1B1 or compare the levels of CYP1B1 in various types of cancer is through immunohistochemical staining for CYP1B1.

A human tissue sample is obtained either through biopsy or surgical removal of a tumour. Scientists generally rely on the services of tissue banks to obtain these samples. With a sample in hand the first step is to fix the sample. This is a process by which the sample is made solid. Through the addition of wax or some other solidifying agent, very thin slices (microtomes) can be obtained for microscopic examination.

Once fixed, a microtome is produced and treated with an antibody against CYP1B1. The antibody will adhere to CYP1B1 and will not adhere to cells that do not express CYP1B1. A second antibody is then prepared with a black or brown stain. The second antibody is an antibody against the first antibody (the CYP1B1 antibody). The sample is then treated with this stained, second antibody. The stained antibody adheres to the CYP1B1 antibody, which in turn is adhering to the CYP1B1 enzyme. In this two-step fashion the CYP1B1 enzymes are stained black or brown (depending on the stain used). The microtome is then prepared with a purple stain that dyes the healthy cells purple to highlight the contrast.

Upon microscopic examination of the microtome an array of black/brown cells and purple cells will be seen. This affords the scientist a visual contrast from which they can both see the presence of the CYP1B1 enzyme and the degree of its expression. This process has allowed scientists to determine that the CYP1B1 enzyme is present in all stages of cancer and all types of cancer that have been tested, while not being present in healthy tissue.

At present no commercially available blood test exists for the detection of CYP1B1 although research aimed at realising a minimally invasive test is underway and described in a later chapter.

CYP1B1: PROBLEM OR SOLUTION?

With a discovery such as CYP1B1 the question quickly gets asked, 'is this intrinsic property of cancer cells part of the problem or part of the solution?' In an attempt to address this question, teams of researchers started investigating the metabolic activity of CYP1B1 and came up with a variety of surprising results.

First among these is the finding that anti-cancer agents such as Docetaxel, Tegafur and Flutamide are metabolised by CYP1B1 *(Rochat B., et al., 2001; Michael M., et al.,*

2005). Furthermore, McFayden et al., have reported that Docetaxel, Ellipticine, Mitoxantrone and Tamoxifen are inactivated by CYP1B1 *(McFadyen MCE, et al., 2004).* These cytotoxic agents are not well targeted to cancer cells, that is, they lack selectivity. Given this, upon initial use they are more toxic to healthy tissue than cancerous tissue until such time as CYP1B1 is overwhelmed by the dosage of the cytotoxic agent. Not the result that one wants when the objective is to kill off cancer cells. In light of these research findings CYP1B1 inhibitors are often administered prior to delivery of the anti-cancer agents that are de-activated by CYP1B1.

Another area of significant research activity is the conversion of estradiol to 4-hydroxyestradiol . This conversion is catalyzed by CYP1B1 *(Hayes, CI, et al., 1996).* Of potential concern here is the carcinogenic and mutagenic properties of 4-hydroxyestradiol *(Zhao Z, et al., 2006).* This has led to speculation that CYP1B1 and its polymorphisms may explain individual differences in breast cancer risk *(Hanna IH, et al., 2000).* Given that CYP1B1 is an intrinsic property of cancer cells rather than healthy cells it has been pointed out that if we are to implicate CYP1B1 in breast cancer it should be for intratumoural metabolism of estradiol *(McFadyen MCE, et al., 1999)* rather than as a causal agent. This, of course, would take CYP1B1 out of the running in terms of breast cancer risk as once CYP1B1 is detectable the breast cancer is present.

CYP1B1 has also been shown to activate a broad array of procarcinogens into environmental carcinogens *(Shimada, T. et al., 1996).* Of significant interest to smokers is the finding that CYP1B1 can convert procarcinogens in tobacco smoke, including benzo[*a*]pyrene (B[*a*]P), into carcinogens. Further to this, tobacco smoke induces

CYP1B1 in the aerodigestive tract including the tongue, oesophagus, colon and lung. This leads researchers to speculate that the induction of CYP1B1 by tobacco smoke may amplify the mutagenic effects of smoke borne carcinogens (*Port, J. et al., 2004*). In stark contrast to these results is the fact that carbon monoxide is a CYP1B1 inhibitor. Given this, one is led to believe that results in practice may be quite different than those obtained under experimental, laboratory conditions.

Metabolism of anti-cancer agents and activation of procarcinogens to carcinogens can certainly cause people to view CYP1B1 with suspicion. It is an intrinsic component of all cancer cells, it diminishes the activity of various anti-cancer agents and can actively transform procarcinogens into carcinogens. This transforming of procarcinogens into carcinogens gets people quite alarmed, but we need to remember that CYP1B1 is confined to cancer cells. We must ask 'how bad can it be if a carcinogen is created within a cancer cell?' The cell is already cancerous! It would be more sensible to focus on what would prevent the cancer in the first instance.

Before we conclude that CYP1B1 is part of the problem we must ask ourselves why does CYP1B1 exist? It has been around for millennia (actually it has been detected in mammals as far back in history as one hundred and fifty million years ago) so what is the survival value of this enzyme? What is the role of CYP1B1?

It is certainly farfetched to think that CYP1B1 has been lurking around all this time waiting for humans to start smoking! It is similarly farfetched to think that it has simply been waiting for humans to invent chemotherapies so that it could render them inactive. By the same token it stretches the imagination to think that CYP1B1 has been quietly biding its time waiting for us to invent and ingest procarcinogens so that it can transform them into carcinogens. Where is the survival value in all of this? The evolutionary longevity of this enzyme would argue that it likely aids in our survival rather than facilitates our demise. Why else would it exist?

Those that argue that CYP1B1 is part of the problem are making the same logical error as those that would have us believe that police are at the root of all crime because they are always present at crime scenes (*Potter G, 2005*).

Perhaps these findings are side effects of CYP1B1 currently operating in an age of industrial, environmental and pharmaceutical chemicals. Perhaps its actual function is far more fundamental to human survival. To arrive at this view one must come to the problem from quite a different perspective.

3.

STILSERENE: A CYP1B1 TARGETED PRODRUG

This works, I know it works. It is frustrating not
to be able to move faster, but we will get there.
I believe that, I really do.

❖ GERRY POTTER, PH.D.

At the Cancer Drug Discovery Group at De Montfort
University in Leicester, England, Professor Potter took a
different tact with respect to CYP1B1. Professor Potter
is a medicinal chemist in the School of Pharmacy at De
Montfort University. Fortuitously, Professor Burke was the
head of the School of Pharmacy while Professor Potter was
Director of the Cancer Drug Discovery Group.

Professor Potter had already successfully designed an
inhibitor, Abiraterone acetate, for the cytochrome P450

enzyme CYP17 when Professor Burke described the CYP1B1 enzyme to him. Potter immediately viewed the specificity of this enzyme as a target for developing cancer therapies - therapies that would be benign until activated by enzymatic reaction - prodrugs.

Upon hearing about the specifics of the hydroxylation action of CYP1B1 on estradiol, Professor Potter started to formulate an approach to realising such a prodrug. Within a week he had designed two distinct prodrugs that could theoretically be activated by CYP1B1. He settled on one of these for development and successfully built the compound.

Unlike conventional chemotherapy this compound was designed to be benign upon entry into the human body and completely targeted to CYP1B1, hence, completely targeted to the cancer cells. The compound, 'Stilserene', is metabolised by the CYP1B1 enzyme to produce a metabolite within the cancer cell that induces apoptosis (programmed cell death) while leaving healthy tissue unharmed – no side effects (*Potter G. et al., 2001*)!

Laboratory testing of Stilserene demonstrated that it was effective at inducing cell death in 95% of the cancer cells tested. This test included cancers that were resistant to other treatments. Stomach, colon, lung, breast and brain cancer cells were all destroyed by Stilserene with no damage to healthy tissue.

This result represents an enormous departure from results with traditional chemotherapy. Traditional chemotherapy is usually as toxic to healthy tissue as it is to cancerous tissue. At best it will be twice as toxic to cancerous tissue as it is to healthy tissue. By comparison Stilserene proved to be over 4,304 times as toxic to cancer cells as healthy tissue and its toxicity was confined within the cancer cell.

Stilserene ushers in a new era of cancer intervention - broadly applicable cancer therapy without debilitating side effects. In light of these results Professor Potter was quoted as saying, "I never believed that cancer was a curable disease. Now, in the light of what we have discovered, I believe that cancer is curable." (*BBC, 2001*).

As news of this new drug reached the public Professor Potter became inundated with pleas for help from all corners of the globe. An example taken from the myriad of letters and emails that he received was published in the local newspaper.

"You are our only hope, says the neatly-typed letter bearing a Bulgarian address. If you do not help us our daughter, our 'beautiful, playful, mischievous,' Lora will die." (*Leicester Mercury, 2003*).

Against this heart-rending backdrop of cries for help the Cancer Drug Discovery Group pressed ahead with the research. A water-soluble version of Stilserene was realised, thereby opening the door for production of a capsule that could be taken orally and easily digested.

Techniques were developed to scale up production of the drug. From the few small crystals realised in the first instance, the team managed to scale the production up to the point that kilograms of the drug could be produced. This opened the door to interest from companies large enough to pursue the enormously costly clinical trials that were needed.

Stilserene has recently been licensed to a pharmaceutical company and is currently being prepared for clinical trials. Wide-spread use of Stilserene is still many, many years away. The Leicester Mercury, a daily newspaper in Leicester that has covered Potter's work, outlines a minimum of seven years up to a maximum of fourteen years before Stilserene is available by prescription. This timeline is not out of line with the FDA's 'new drug development timeline'. The FDA timeline outlines a minimum of five years, a maximum of twenty years and an average of eight and one half years for a new drug to successfully travel through the approval process prior to being available by prescription (for more information please see the timetable for new drug approval from www.fda.gov.

In the face of this time scale and with the countless pleas for his help in mind Professor Potter was quoted as saying "This works, I know it works. It is frustrating not to be able to move faster, but we will get there. I believe that, I really do." (*Leicester Mercury, 2003*).

4.

DISCOVERY OF FOOD-BASED, CANCER PRODRUGS

I never believed that cancer was a curable disease. Now, in the light of what we have discovered, I believe that cancer is curable.

❖ GERRY POTTER, PH.D.

The Stilserene experience caused Professor Potter to re-examine the role of CYP1B1. Since Stilserene was so effective across such a broad array of cancers could CYP1B1 be a rescue mechanism to rid the body of cancer? A defence mechanism to save us from malignancies? Perhaps, as Professor Potter points out, the question to ask is not 'why do we get cancer' but rather 'why don't we all get cancer?' (*Potter, G, 2005*). If CYP1B1 is a rescue mechanism perhaps this is the reason why we don't all get cancer!

This idea was bolstered by the fact that the chemical structure of Stilserene struck Professor Potter as being very similar to natural compounds that he was familiar with. If CYP1B1 was a rescue mechanism then it would follow that compounds should occur in nature that are metabolised by CYP1B1, in a manner similar to Stilserene, to rid the body of cancer. More specifically, compounds should occur in food that are metabolised by CYP1B1 to the same result as metabolism of Stilserene because food, as a source of these compounds, would ensure that CYP1B1 would have the material that it needed to rid the body of cancer making this rescue mechanism viable.

This re-evaluation of the role of CYP1B1 drove the search for a natural compound that would behave, in the face of CYP1B1, as a prodrug with resultant anti-cancer properties. This took the research into a very interesting new direction.

THE RESVERATROL STORY

Concurrent with the design and testing of Stilserene considerable attention was being paid to research into what became known as the French paradox. The French diet involves a lot of fatty foods such as cheeses, red meats and rich sauces, yet the French do not seem to suffer from high cholesterol and consequent heart problems to the same degree as some of their European neighbours. Researchers had closed in on resveratrol, a natural compound found in the skins of grapes and French red wines, as the dietary mechanism that accounted for this paradox as red wine is a typical complement to a meal in France.

In the quest for a natural compound that would behave like Stilserene, resveratrol came to the attention of Professor Potter and his research team. Resveratrol had been shown to have cancer preventative properties (Jang, M. et al, 1997; Jang, M. et al, 1999). More importantly resveratrol is a stilbene with a chemical structure similar to that of Stilserene (stilbenes are hydrocarbons, $C_{14}H_{12}$, that are used in the production of dyes and synthetic estrogens). In addition, resveratrol is a phytoestrogen that is structurally similar to estradiol. It was reasoned that given this structural similarity resveratrol may undergo aromatic hydroxylation by CYP1B1 in the same manner as estradiol. If this hydroxylation took place at the same site in resveratrol as it does in estradiol a very beneficial metabolite would be realised (*Potter, G, et al, 2002*).

If this proved to be the case this would support Professor Potter's contention that CYP1B1 was a "rescue enzyme" to activate certain dietary compounds into anti-cancer agents within the confines of cancer cells - a dietary mechanism to protect the body against cancer. Resveratrol seemed like the right natural compound to investigate.

Experiments were conducted that determined that in the presence of CYP1B1 resveratrol is converted into piceatannol, another stilbene structure with known anti-cancer properties (*Ferrigni, N. 1984*). This result outlined a molecular level mechanism whereby a dietary compound could act as a natural prodrug being activated into an anticancer agent within the cancer cell by the CYP1B1 enzyme (*Potter, G, et al, 2002*). From this research we now understand the following natural prodrug mechanism:

benign, natural compound	+	metabolising enzyme	=	anticancer agent
resveratrol	+	CYP1B1	=	piceatannol

The beauty of the mechanism is that it all takes place within the confines of the cancer cell. The anticancer agent is produced within the cancer cell and operates exclusively within the cancer cell so that healthy tissue remains totally unaffected. This is exactly what one wants in a therapeutic intervention – selectivity -a natural therapeutic intervention that selectively targets cancer cells.

INITIAL TESTING ON A VARIETY OF CANCERS

Leicester is home to the largest tissue bank in Great Britain. This proximity is a great boon to the cancer research conducted at De Montfort University, home of Professor Potter's Cancer Drug Discovery Group. With the bioactivation of resveratrol to piceatannol by CYP1B1 illuminated, research was carried out to test the efficacy and selectivity of the mechanism on cancer cell lines. As was done with Stilserene, tests were conducted on various cancer cell lines concurrent with tests on healthy tissue. As was found with Stilserene, no harm was done to the healthy tissue while apoptosis (programmed cell death) was induced in the cancer cells. In short, the healthy tissue was untouched while the cancer cells died.

There was, however, one critical difference between the results for Stilserene and resveratrol. Resveratrol was effective in killing cancer cells at exceptionally low doses, but as the dose increased a self-inhibiting effect was observed –

higher doses of resveratrol inhibited the activity of CYP1B1 thereby shutting off the metabolic activity of CYP1B1 and leaving the cancer cells unharmed (see Figure 1).

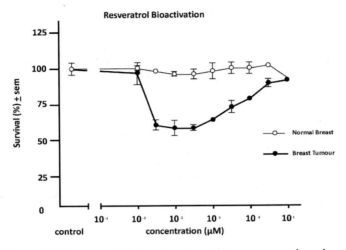

Figure 1. Resveratrol bioactivation. (Figure reproduced with the kind permission of Prof. Gerry Potter).

This figure shows that resveratrol is not activated in the normal breast cells where CYP1B1 is not present but is activated in the breast tumour cells where CYP1B1 is present. As the concentration of resveratrol increased (x axis or bottom axis) the survival rate of the breast tumour cells (y axis or side axis) quickly returned to 100%. With resveratrol, not only does the effectiveness at killing cancer cells go to zero, CYP1B1 is concurrently inhibited so that it cannot metabolise any other compounds that could potentially kill the cells. This effect, although scientifically interesting, makes resveratrol of minimal use as a potential cancer therapeutic as it is excessively difficult to determine how much would be appropriate for anyone wishing to use it.

THE QUEST FOR FOOD-BASED PRODRUGS

The resveratrol experience stimulated a search for additional food-based compounds that would behave as natural, anticancer prodrugs. If, as the resveratrol research seemed to indicate, the functional role of CYP1B1 is to rid the body of cancer cells, through metabolism of food-based, natural compounds into anticancer agents, then it would stand to reason that similar compounds should exist.

An understanding of the metabolic activity of CYP1B1 provided the clues as to the chemical structure to look for. This then left the problem of where to look. Texts on traditional plant-based medicines, plant-based diets from cultures with a low incidence of cancer and historic texts on herbalism served to guide the search.

Researchers began extensive analysis of fruits, berries, vegetables and herbs in the quest for additional natural compounds that would behave like Stilserene and resveratrol. The search has been productive. To date there are over twenty natural, food-based compounds that have been discovered, analysed and tested. They form a collection of hydrophilic and lipophilic compounds. All have this defining characteristic of being metabolised by CYP1B1 into a metabolite with anticancer function. They are all secondary plant metabolites: phytoalexins.

5.
SALVESTROLS

Let food be your medicine and medicine be
your food.

❖ HIPPOCRATES, 400 BC

Professor Potter coined the term "Salvestrols" for this new class of phytonutrients. The term Salvestrols is a derivation of the Latin 'salvia' (to save), the sage herb, which was a medieval herbal remedy.

As more salvestrols have been discovered the understanding has advanced. From analysis of these salvestrols it is predicted that the class of salvestrols will ultimately include over fifty phytonutrients. The quest continues.

WHAT ARE SALVESTROLS?

Salvestrols are a new class of phytonutrients that have a pharmacological definition rather than a chemical definition. They are defined by the action of the metabolites produced when they are metabolised by the CYP1B1 enzyme in cancer cells. Simply put, salvestrols are food-based compounds that are metabolised by CYP1B1 to produce metabolites that are anticancer agents. These anticancer agents suppress tumour growth by killing the cancer cells.

Salvestrols are also part of the plants immune system. They are phytoalexins. They are elicited, in a pathogen specific manner, by invading fungi or pathogens to inhibit the action of the invading pathogen.

Salvestrols do not fall neatly into any of the existing classes of phytonutrients. Resveratrol, for example, is both a polyphenol and a phytoestrogen. Of the salvestrols discovered to date some are antioxidants, some are polyphenols, some are phytoestrogens, others do not fall into any of these categories while still others fall into more than one of these categories.

Focusing on the fact that some salvestrols fall into these categories misses the point. They are not providing their anticancer properties due to their being an antioxidant, polyphenol or phytoestrogen. They are providing their anticancer activity through their metabolism by CYP1B1 and specifically through their metabolism to an anticancer agent within the confines of the cancer cell. This is the central, defining feature of salvestrols.

WHAT SETS SALVESTROLS APART: SELECTIVITY

When we show up at our doctor's office with a broken arm we anticipate that the arm will be set in a cast or brace. We expect a selective response to the problem that we present with. If we come away from the doctor's office with casts or braces covering a broad array of body parts that may or may not include the affected arm we are not likely to pay this doctor a return visit!

Similarly, when we present at our doctor's office with disease we anticipate that a therapy will be prescribed that will deal with the diseased cells while leaving the healthy cells unharmed. Again we anticipate a selective response.

The selectively of potential therapies, whether they are synthetic drugs or natural products, is determined through a specific series of experiments. Tests are conducted on healthy cells and diseased cells. An array of test receptacles will be arranged, with an equal number of cells in each, such that individual tests can be conducted on the healthy cells and the diseased cells at a large variety of dose levels of the therapeutic agent in question. A minimal dose is chosen to start the testing and this dose is then increased logarithmically such that the next highest dose is always 10 times the dose level of the previous test.

The concentration is increased in this fashion until a dose is reached that is beyond that which is achievable in the human body. In each receptacle the percentage of cells that are killed are recorded for both the healthy cells and the diseased cells. For each type of cell the dose at which 50% of the cells die is recorded. A ratio of the doses at this level is then derived and used as a metric of the selectivity of the therapy. A selectively of 1 essentially means that the therapeutic agent is as toxic to healthy tissue as it is to diseased tissue. The higher the selectivity number the more selective the therapy is in targeting the diseased cells.

From a practical point of view one must look at the amount of healthy tissue in the human body compared to the amount of diseased tissue. When an agent with a selectivity of 1 is introduced into the human body it will kill healthy tissue with the same propensity as it will kill diseased tissue, but, it will run into a lot more healthy tissue to kill than it will diseased tissue. Consequently, much more healthy tissue will be killed. This is why the selectivity of the agent is so important.

Selectivity testing has been done on a broad array of salvestrols and the results are extremely good. Salvestrol research commenced with two salvestrols: S40 and S31G. The central difference between these salvestrols is that S31G is lipophilic, that is, it can diffuse through tissue very readily. It can pass through the blood-brain barrier and get to tissues that non-lipophilic compounds would have more difficulty reaching. S31G is also found in very few plants, such as, a variety of tangerine, olives and asparagus. A newly discovered subclass of salvestrols, the 5 series, has also recently been tested.

The following table highlights the selectivity of a classic chemotherapy and contrasts this with the selectivity of a variety of salvestrols including the original two plus a few from the newly discovered 5 series.

Compound:	Classification:	Selectivity score:
Methotrexate	chemotherapy	= 1
S40	salvestrol	= 10
S31G	salvestrol	= 22
S52	salvestrol	= 32
S54	salvestrol	= 1,250
Stilserene	synthetic salvestrol	= 4,304
S55	salvestrol	= 23,000

The selectivity of salvestrols represents a significant improvement over classical chemotherapy. The selectivity values for salvestrols from the 5 series, such as those for S55 are beyond those obtained for the Stilserene drug that Professor Potter originally developed. Nature has had a long time to get this right!

The selectivity that we see with salvestrols comes from the fact that they are targeted to the CYP1B1 enzyme. They are acting like natural prodrugs with their cancer fighting being confined within the cancer cells. The healthy tissue remains unharmed. This is an enormous step forward from conventional cancer therapies and is a distinguishing feature of salvestrols.

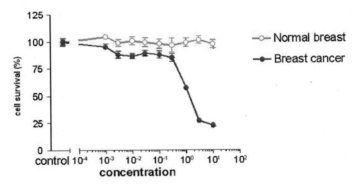

Figure 2. Salvestrol bioactivation. (Figure reproduced with the kind permission of Prof. Gerry Potter).

Figure 2 highlights the selectivity of salvestrols. Cells from a healthy, normal breast do not contain CYP1B1. Consequently they do not activate salvestrols and remain totally unharmed, that is, none of these cells die at the salvestrol concentrations shown in this figure. In contrast the breast cancer cells do contain CYP1B1 and as we can see CYP1B1 activates the salvestrols and the breast cancer cells start to die off. In contrast to what we observed with resveratrol, as the dose of this salvestrol increases the percentage of cancer cells dying increases. This is exactly what a targeted therapy should look like.

SALVESTROLS ROLE IN PLANTS

In order to fully understand salvestrols it is necessary to understand their role in the plants that produce them. Plants are subject to attack by various pathogens, primarily fungi. These attacks generally occur late in the ripening phase. These pathogens usually attack the skin of the fruit and/or the roots of the plant. In response to these attacks plants have evolved a defence mechanism and that defence mechanism is salvestrols.

In plants, salvestrols are produced, primarily, on an 'if and when needed' basis. When the plant is attacked salvestrols are elicited at the site of the infection: the skin of the fruit or the root of the plant. From here the salvestrol penetrates the pathogen.

It is known that fungi, like humans and other life forms, house various cytochrome P450 enzymes. The destruction of the pathogen is brought about by metabolism of the salvestrol into a antifungal agent, within the fungi, by a cytochrome P450 enzyme in fungi that has similar metabolic activity to the CYP1B1 enzyme in cancer cells. Salvestrols are natural antifungal agents.

CYP1B1 may be an adaptation that enables us to borrow the plant's defence mechanism and make it part of our own defences. The plant produces salvestrols that enter the invading pathogen and induce its death through their metabolism by a CYP enzyme in fungi. We eat the salvestrol rich plant and those same salvestrols enter our cancer cells and induce their death through metabolism by CYP1B1. In addition, the salvestrols will enter any fungi that they encounter in the human body and act as natural antifungal agents in the same way as they do in the plants from which they were obtained. In these situations, it appears that what is good for the plant is good for the gardener.

As mentioned previously there are many different salvestrols. What has recently come to light is the fact that different pathogens can induce production of different salvestrols. This effect can take place within the same plant when facing attack from multiple pathogens (*Daniels A, 2006*). This result opens up the fascinating prospect of stimulating plants for production of salvestrols in general, and for production of specific salvestrols or specific combinations of salvestrols in particular, through the selective introduction of pathogens.

LINK BETWEEN CANCER AND DIET

We have all come across statements asserting that there is a link between diet and cancer. The World Health Organisation has embarked on a world-wide campaign to increase fruit and vegetable consumption in an effort to stem the rise of disease. Following this lead a variety of governmental health departments have initiated their own campaigns. (A sampling from these various campaigns is outlined in Appendix 2).

Whereas the campaign to increase fruit and vegetable consumption makes intuitive sense, and is supported by epidemiological work, the campaigners fail to explain how these dietary changes should assist us. In the absence of such an explanation these campaigns run the risk of being taken lightly or dismissed altogether.

THE SALVESTROL CONCEPT: ONE MECHANISM EXPLAINED

The work of Professors Potter and Burke has converged on the first molecular level explanation of a mechanism for linking diet and cancer. A mechanism that can explain how fruit and vegetable consumption can prevent and treat cancer. This mechanism has become known as the Salvestrol Concept.

There are three components to the salvestrol concept. These are salvestrols, the CYP1B1 enzyme and the metabolites that are formed by the metabolism of salvestrols by CYP1B1.

This concept is illustrated as follows:

Phytonutrients found in fruit & vegetables	+	Enzyme intrinsic to cancer cells	=	Apoptosis – cell death
Salvestrols	+	CYP1B1	=	Anticancer agent

It is often reported that cancer cells are forming in the human body on a continual basis. For a person with a diet rich in organic fruits and vegetables we can anticipate the following scenario:

Salvestrols are taken through fruit and vegetable consump-tion and enter our cells. The salvestrols pass through healthy tissue with no consequence. As they enter a cancer cell they encounter the CYP1B1 enzyme. CYP1B1 metabolises the salvestrol, transforming it into an anticancer agent within the cancer cell. This anticancer agent, the metabolite, then initiates the cascade of processes that result in the death of the cancer cell – apoptosis or programmed cell death. The healthy cells remain healthy and the cancer cells die.

This same mechanism is operating regardless of wheth-er the cell is precancerous, part of a primary tumour or part of the metastases of that primary tumour. The salves-trol mechanism is, therefore, as important for prevention as it is for treatment of full-blown cancers.

From this perspective we would anticipate that when adequate levels of salvestrols are ingested, this mechanism would deal with the cancer cells that are formed as they arise. Conversely as the level of salvestrol intake decreases the number of cancer cells left to flourish would likely in-crease.

A central message to take from this mechanism is that dietary change can have enormous and long-term conse-quences for the improvement of your health. Incorporation of a large amount of organic fruits and vegetables into one's diet represents a significant step towards good health.

AN INTERESTING IMPLICATION

Tumours are a mixture of cancer cells and healthy cells. When we look through a microscope at a tissue sample that has been stained to reveal the CYP1B1 enzyme we do not simply see a black or brown mass. The black or brown stained cells (the cancer cells) are interspersed with purple stained cells (the healthy cells).

The Salvestrol Concept outlines a highly targeted mechanism. Salvestrols only become lethal to the cell once metabolised by the CYP1B1 enzyme. Consequently they are only lethal to the cancer cells. An implication of using such a highly targeted therapy is that over time the salvestrols selectively kill the cancer cells within the tumour and leave the healthy cells unharmed. The result can be a benign mass of healthy cells left behind. Such a benign mass can, upon external prodding, remain disconcerting as it will still present as a lump. To alleviate the concern of one with such a lump a biopsy may be necessary to prove that the cancer has been eradicated and the remaining lump is actually a benign collection of healthy tissue.

6.
WHY IS CANCER SO PREVALENT?

There has to be a significant change in the way
that we approach food, in the way we grow food
and the way that we see our diet.

❖ ANTHONY DANIELS

With this elegant mechanism for ridding the body of cancer cells one might ask 'why is cancer so prevalent' and 'why is the prognosis so poor for those suffering from this disease?' From the perspective of this salvestrol mechanism (salvestrol + CYP1B1 = anticancer metabolite) there would be four main factors that come to mind.

First, and most importantly would be a very serious depletion in the salvestrol levels in our diet. We know from the reporting of the World Health Organisation that more than half of all cancer cases occur in the developing world as opposed to the underdeveloped world. Diet likely plays a significant role here.

Second, and significant in its own right would be exposure to inhibitors of the CYP1B1 enzyme. If the CYP1B1 enzyme is inhibited it cannot perform its role metabolising salvestrols.

Thirdly, and to a much less extent than the first two factors, polymorphisms of CYP1B1 likely play a role.

Finally, the levels of CYP1B1 that are expressed within an individual's cancer cells will relate to the efficiency of the salvestrol mechanism.

DEPLETION OF SALVESTROLS

When Professor Potter and his research group set off to find salvestrols they analysed thousands of fruit, vegetable and herb samples. Through this analysis they discovered that salvestrols were present in very small amounts and often not at all in produce found in the local supermarket while much of the organic produce had salvestrols in abundance. In short, they found that our typical western food supply is desperately deficient in salvestrols.

MODERN FARMING PRACTICES

To begin to understand the depletion of salvestrols in our diet we need to look at the influence of modern farming practices. In the 1700s mechanisation was starting to influence farming. Monoculture farming (the growing of a single crop variety over a large area of land) was introduced to take full advantage of advances in mechanised harvesting. Crops that grow at the same rate and to the same height are more amenable to mechanised harvesting.

These efficiencies came at a cost. When a single variety is grown over a large area the entire crop can be lost due to a specific insect infestation, fungal infection or weed infestation. All of the plants have the same vulnerability. To combat crop devastation herbicides, pesticides and fungicides were introduced to keep these various infestations at bay. The result was consistent, perfect looking produce to take to market.

This perfect looking produce, however, was severely depleted in salvestrols. Salvestrols are part of the plants defence against pathogens. As such, if the plant is not subject to pathogens because agricultural chemicals are used to keep the crop artificially free of pathogens, the plants do not receive any signal to produce salvestrols (*Magee, JB, et al,. 2002*). Consequently they do not end up in our food.

Organic produce is the way to avoid this problem. Organically grown produce contains much higher levels of salvestrols and is also free of pesticide, fungicide and herbicide residue. Research has indicated that the level of salvestrols in organic produce is up to 30 times higher than in produce produced through modern farming practices (*Burke MD, 2006*). Incorporating as much organic produce as possible into one's diet will help to increase one's benefit from salvestrols. Utilisation of the whole food will further assist with increasing the levels of salvestrols as they are most abundant in the skins of the fruit or vegetable or in the roots. Incorporating 'smoothies' into one's diet is an easy way of utilising the whole food.

RIPENING PHASE OF THE PRODUCE

Our perfect looking food that appears in our supermarkets is no longer exclusively from local market gardens. Our fruits and vegetables may come from many different continents to ensure that we are offered everything that we may desire on a year round basis.

Salvestrols are generally produced late in the ripening phase as this is when the plant is most vulnerable to attack. Produce is typically picked well before the ripening phase so that it will be ready when it reaches far off grocery stores. Again this affords the plant no opportunity to produce salvestrols. Purchasing locally produced organic produce or having your own fruit and vegetable garden are excellent ways of ensuring that the produce has had a chance to ripen on the vine.

HISTORIC VERSUS NEWER PLANT VARIETIES

A further impediment to salvestrols in our food supply comes from the introduction of newer varieties of fruits and vegetables. People have become accustomed to sweet tasting food. A look at the list of ingredients on items in the grocery store will confirm this – sugar is added to many, many foods. To meet this buyer preference growers have developed new varieties of fruits and vegetables that have a sweeter taste.

Salvestrols often have a sharp and bitter taste. Selecting for sweetness in production of a new variety often means selecting against salvestrol production. Consequently, many of these newer varieties do not produce salvestrols or produce them in minute quantities. The sweetness was obtained at the expense of the salvestrols. With salvestrols lacking in these varieties it becomes necessary to use artificial fungicides to protect them, further aggravating the situation.

A recent study looking at health promoting phytonutrients in apples grown conventionally and organically and including one heritage variety illustrates many of these points. The study shows that organically grown apples contain much higher levels of health promoting phytonutrients than apples grown conventionally. Further to this, the study shows that the peel of the apple contains higher levels than the flesh. However, most importantly the study shows that the heritage apple contained more health promoting phytonutrients and in much higher levels, through both the peel and the flesh, than any of the other apples (*Li N, 2009*). Newer varieties may not be delivering the nutrition that our forefathers enjoyed. When possible, one should try to include the older varieties in one's diet.

FOOD PROCESSING

Food processing can also lead to depletion of salvestrols in our food. For example, cranberries are a good source of salvestrols, yet when cranberry juices are tested they often contain no salvestrols. The reason is that the juices are put through special filters that extract sharp and bitter tasting compounds so that the finished product will taste sweeter without the need to add extra sugar. As salvestrols are often sharp tasting they are filtered out along with a host of other compounds. The result is a clear "100% fruit juice" product with diminished nutritional value. The unfiltered organic juices are a better buy for salvestrol content.

A related effect from food processing is found in the production of olive oil. Olives are a good source of salvestrols. As you will remember salvestrols are elicited on the skins of the fruit as this is the site of assault from pathogens. Historically olive oil was produced using a stone grinding mill. The stones would not only squeeze the olives they would also tear the skins and flesh apart releasing into the oil a host of compounds buried within the cells. The resultant oil was cloudy and a sediment would build on the bottom of the container. Historically the olives were also grown without use of pesticides, fungicides and herbicides. The result was an oil that was rich in salvestrols.

Modern production of olive oil involves cold pressing and filtering. The cold pressing leaves the skins intact thereby releasing very little of the salvestrols into the oil. What does get released into the oil gets filtered out to provide the consumer with the perfectly clear oil that they are used to. Once again nutrition suffers. There are still growers that produce olive oils in the traditional manner. Search out a supplier of olive oil that uses organically grown olives that are stone ground and unfiltered. These can be quite expensive but reasonably priced supplies do exist.

This situation is mirrored in the wine industry. As we found out in an earlier chapter resveratrol is found in the skin of grapes. Resveratrol is found in French wines, pinot noirs in particular, but not to the same degree in New World wines. The difference is twofold. First the French prefer to grow their grapes without the use of fungicides, pesticides, etc. Second they crush the grapes and ferment the wine with the crushed grapes. As alcohol is produced through fermentation the resveratrol is released from the grape skins and enters the liquid. In New World wine production, the grapes are crushed and the resultant juice is fermented. The skins and pulp are discarded prior to fermentation. This process affords no opportunity for the alcohol to release the resveratrol from the grape skins as the grape skins are no longer available by the time the alcohol is being produced.

SUMMERHILL PYRAMID WINERY – A NEW WORLD EXCEPTION

An analysis of the polyphenolic content of grape pomace obtained from Summerhill Pyramid Winery in Kelowna, British Columbia, Canada (www.summerhill.bc.ca) was carried out. Summerhill, under the direction of Steve Cipes, is an organic vineyard. Pomace samples were obtained from a variety of white wines, red wines and both red and white ice wines. Pomace is the pulpy material left behind during the wine making process. A wide variety of polyphenolics were tested for. The results indicated that a high, total polyphenolic content was found for both white wine varieties and red wine varieties with the red wine varieties having much higher polyphenolic content than the white wine varieties. The ice wines, both white and red had much higher polyphenolic content than pomace from any of the wines that were harvested earlier. The red ice wine has much higher polyphenolic content than the white, ice wine. In essence the results can be depicted as follows:

Total polyphenolic content of wine pomace samples
Red ice wine > White ice wine > Red wine > White wine

These results point to the benefits of organic growing. Polyphenolic levels and salvestrol levels (salvestrols are a subset of polyphenolic plant compounds) will be high when the plants are grown organically. These results also serve as an example of the benefits of harvesting late in the ripening phase as with the ice wines that are harvested at the very end of the season. These late harvest grapes have the highest polyphenolic content. Finally, these results indicate that new world wine production can have very high polyphenolic, and hence salvestrol content, when the growing is organic and the production method includes fermentation with the crushed grapes (*Pruh'homme A, 2009*). As Steve Cipes of Summerhill Winery puts it "*This research shows that using traditional processes and using organic grapes makes a wine that is superior for our health, as well as being good for the environment. It shows that you don't have to use chemicals to make a great wine. I have always instinctively known that but it is great to have the science now to back it up!.*"

The combination of modern farming practices, lengthy transportation times, introduction of new varieties and food processing leave us with a food supply that is seriously deficient in salvestrols. Without salvestrols in the diet the CYP1B1 enzyme cannot protect us from cancer. We could learn something from the example set by Summerhill Pyramid Winery!

CYP1B1 INHIBITION

The CYP1B1 enzyme can react with many different substances aside from salvestrols. The lifecycle of the CYP1B1 enzyme is around three days. That is, each molecule of

CYP1B1 enzyme is replaced by a new one roughly every three days.

Some of the substances that CYP1B1 can encounter are inhibitors of this enzyme. Once one of these inhibitory substances binds with CYP1B1, the enzyme is unfortunately prevented from metabolising and activating Salvestrols. So anyone who has a CYP1B1 inhibitor in their body will have the inhibitors and the salvestrols competing for the CYP1B1 enzyme. The competition will depend, at least in part, on the relative levels of both the inhibitors and the salvestrols in the body as well as their respective affinity for CYP1B1. Suffice it to say that when CYP1B1 inhibitors are in the body one will forego the full benefit that the salvestrols could deliver.

The inhibition from some inhibitors will last the full life cycle of the enzyme. It is important that people seeking benefit from salvestrols reduce or, preferably, eliminate their exposure to inhibitors of CYP1B1 to give the salvestrols their best chance of being activated so that cancer cell death can occur. Powerful inhibitors of CYP1B1 include carbon monoxide (e.g. in tobacco smoke), vitamin B17 (e.g. in the kernels of apricots and bitter almonds - also encountered as amygdalin or laetrile), and certain agrochemical fungicides.

The agrochemical fungicides are doubly problematic. When used on crops they impair the plant's production of salvestrols. The plants will only produce the salvestrols in abundance when under attack from pathogens. Inside the human body these same fungicides inhibit the CYP1B1 enzyme so that one cannot take full advantage of any salvestrols that may be in one's system. This is certainly not an ideal scenario.

Agrochemical fungicides are of course used in agriculture but they are also used elsewhere which makes their avoidance difficult. Fungicides can be used on golf courses, public park areas, in new carpeting, dandruff shampoos, house paints and can be added to the cleaning agents used when heating ductwork is cleaned.

CYP1B1 POLYMORPHISMS

Salvestrols are metabolised by the CYP1B1 enzyme. The metabolite brings about a cascade of events within the cancer cells that induce their death. CYP1B1 exists, predominantly, in its standard or 'wild' form. However, there are four main versions of CYP1B1 (*Li DN., et al, 2000*). Up to 50% of some populations inherit (from their parents) one of these four versions of the CYP1B1 enzyme - this is called a genetic polymorphism.

These polymorphisms have been shown to have different ability to metabolise salvestrols. Research indicates that the scale of this reduction in activity is not likely to be huge. (For a detailed discussion of polymorphisms see Professor Dan Burke's article in the Winter 2006 issue of Health Action Magazine – *Burke D., 2006*).

It is important to stress here that although people with a rare inherited type of glaucoma (primary congenital glaucoma) tend to have versions of CYP1B1 that are totally inactive, this disease occurs almost exclusively in Southeast Asia (the Indian sub-continent) and parts of the Middle East. The type of glaucoma that vastly predominates in Western countries confers no loss of CYP1B1 activity. Primary congenital glaucoma affects approximately 1 person in every 10,000.

LEVELS OF CYP1B1 EXPRESSION

The levels of CYP1B1 that are expressed in cancer cells will vary from cancer to cancer and from person to person. Of greatest interest is the variability from person to person. When tumour tissue samples from a specific type of cancer are compared across individuals a range of CYP1B1 expression levels are observed. Some will express an abundance of CYP1B1 while others will express relatively small amounts. The expression level will certainly relate to how well an individual will respond to salvestrols. The more CYP1B1 there is to metabolise the salvestrols the better the individual will respond. With this said it should be noted that differences in the expression level may be due to differences in the laboratory methods for detecting and measuring CYP1B1 levels.

CYP1B1 results from a variety of induction pathways, that is, processes that lead to the production of CYP1B1. The science behind these various induction pathways is beyond our current discussion. However, suffice it to say that those people that are expressing very low levels of CYP1B1 will be experiencing some interruption of one or more of these induction pathways. One way of increasing the production of CYP1B1 is to ensure that one is taking the recommended dietary allowance (RDA) of biotin (vitamin H) in one's diet as biotin has been shown to induce production of CYP1B1.

7.
NATURE'S DEFENCE

Man is a food-dependent creature. If you don't
feed him, he will die. If you feed him improperly,
part of him will die.

❖ EMANUEL CHERASKIN, M.D., D.M.D.

When the work of cancer researchers is reported in the mainstream press an enormous response from the public often follows. The discovery of salvestrols and formulation of the Salvestrol Concept was done against a continual backdrop of requests for help from cancer sufferers, their friends and loved ones looking for assistance. During this time members of the research team, like all of us, were confronted with loved ones and friends being diagnosed with cancer.

Given that food forms the foundation of the Salvestrol Concept the initial response to the public was formulation of a dietary recommendation: point them to those organically produced foods that are high in salvestrols! Professor Potter put together what has become known as the Green and Red Diet, a copy of which is reproduced with his kind permission in Appendix 3.

The research team was convinced that nature provided a natural, food-based prodrug in the form of salvestrols. CYP1B1 served as the rescue enzyme to metabolise those salvestrols into anticancer agents and rid the body of cancer cells in the same fashion as the synthetic drug Stilserene. The research team continued to explore various herbs and foods that had historically been viewed as having health benefits.

Through these efforts the team discovered that artichoke was a very rich source of very potent salvestrols. Artichokes have a great amount of surface area for salvestrols to collect because they are made up of many, many small leaves. Salvestrols make up a remarkable four percent of the dried weight of artichokes. Given the potency of the salvestrols in question and the abundance of them in artichokes the research team was excited about this find.

Fortuitously a pamphlet came through the mail to Professor Potter's residence advertising the products of a local Leicester company: The Herbal Apothecary. What struck Potter's eye was an artichoke extract product – a potential source of salvestrols! With that a telephone call was placed to The Herbal Apothecary and a meeting set up with the Managing Director, Anthony Daniels.

ANTHONY DANIELS

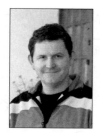

Anthony Daniels is a mechanical engineer by training and a recognised authority within the herbal industry for his innovative techniques and his development of novel products. During the past fifteen years he has developed his expertise in the traditional uses of herbs and plants. He is well recognised for his expertise in herb and plant extraction methods and technologies.

Anthony has pioneered unique environmental botanical technology for the conversion of oil waste into a non-hazardous biomass. Subsequently he developed a unique botanical technology to replace the use of agrochemicals in banana growing with equally effective botanical extracts.

As a founder and Managing Director of The Herbal Apothecary Anthony developed a world-wide set of contracts within the food industry, the herbalist community and organic growers. This background proved to be enormously important for furthering Professor Potter's work.

NEED FOR A SALVESTROL SUPPLEMENT

The Salvestrol Concept points out the overwhelming benefits of a diet with abundant, organically produced fruits and vegetables. With such a diet one will take a daily intake of salvestrols that will aid the body in ridding itself of cancer cells as they arise. This diet is likely what accounts for the lower rates of cancer in those societies that still live largely on traditionally grown fruits and vegetables.

Cancer cells are developing all the time and with such a diet the salvestrols, in concert with the CYP1B1 rescue enzyme, can keep pace with this development and help prevent the development of full blown cancers.

The problem facing the developed world is somewhat different. Cancer is rampant in our societies. Intake of salvestrols from the Western diet is random at best. Even those that have switched to a purely organic food supply can still have a diminished salvestrol intake if the varieties of fruit and vegetables that they are eating are from recently developed varieties developed for sweeter taste. On top of this people have only a modest knowledge of salvestrols and next to no knowledge of the inhibitors that can interfere with the rescue enzyme's ability to metabolise salvestrols.

In short, the Western world is dealing with a vast array of full blown cancers at the same time as it is dealing with a host of lifestyle and workplace risk factors that feed this epidemic. A simple shift in diet may not be sufficient for those already at risk or fighting active disease.

DEVELOPMENT OF A SALVESTROL FOOD SUPPLEMENT

On the strength of their discussions regarding the depletion of salvestrols in the food supply, Professor Potter and Anthony Daniels agreed that a food supplement was needed and formed Nature's Defence (UK) Ltd., as the vehicle to develop it and further the science. Nature's Defence was realised in January of 2004 with a set of corporate articles that directed profits back to salvestrol research.

Anthony Daniels took over the task of determining which fruits and vegetables were the best sources of salvestrols. Thousands of foods were screened. This proved to be a particularly laborious task. There are over five hundred varieties of tangerines and fewer than five actually produce salvestrols! Nevertheless a candidate list of fruits providing salvestrols was found.

This of course left the question of where in the world could vast amounts of organically grown fruits be obtained to produce a reliable supply of salvestrols - they were not likely to come from the United Kingdom in quantities that would sustain production of a food supplement. Anthony Daniels utilised his contacts throughout the world-wide food processing industry and was able to focus the search on the best prospects.

With sources of abundant fruit found the final hurdle to overcome was how to extract the salvestrols so that they could ensure that each capsule would contain the amount of salvestrols that their research had dictated would be helpful to people wishing to utilise salvestrols. Anthony utilised the knowledge that he had gathered in his quest for a replacement of the agrochemicals in the banana growing industry to pioneer a carbon dioxide (CO_2) extraction method for isolating salvestrols from the thousands of phytonutrients found in fruit. With these obstacles overcome Nature's Defence was in a position to bring these discoveries to those that needed them to aid in their fight with disease.

MAXIMISING THE EFFECTIVENESS OF SALVESTROLS

Salvestrols and the CYP1B1 rescue enzyme represent truly remarkable discoveries. However, if one is going to maximise the effectiveness of salvestrols for improvement of one's health there are a few things that are advisable.

DIET

First among these is a change in diet. These discoveries point to the value of foods grown organically. Aside from the specific value of salvestrols these discoveries also remind us that there is still much to learn about the various constituents of the foods we eat – more beneficial compounds will be discovered in these foods as research continues. Incorporating a large amount of organic fruits, berries, vegetables and herbs into one's diet will help to maximise the effectiveness of the salvestrols, provide you with additional salvestrols and set you on a dietary path that will be beneficial for the rest of your life.

Not everyone lives in a community that is well supplied with organic produce. Incorporation of organic produce into the diet, to the degree possible given local supply, will represent a great dietary improvement. Augmenting local supply with your own garden is an excellent way of ensuring the nutritional value of what you eat.

Maximising your intake of organic produce relative to your intake of non organic produce will dramatically reduce your exposure to agrochemicals. Since many agrochemicals are known to inhibit human enzymes, including CYP1B1, this dietary change is very, very worthwhile.

When you are unable to obtain organic produce soak your non organic produce in acidified water (5 – 10% vinegar) for about an hour. This will help to remove the harmful chemicals from the produce, which is very beneficial, but it will do nothing to increase the nutritional properties of the non organic produce.

EXERCISE

Second among these is exercise. Taking some modest exercise each day will help to keep the body well oxygenated. There are a variety of reasons why this is advantageous, but within the confines of our discussion suffice it to say that a good supply of oxygen is important for the CYP1B1 rescue enzyme to perform its role effectively and efficiently. Hyperbaric oxygen therapy can also be used to ensure that the body is kept well oxygenated and CYP1B1 has the oxygen it needs for efficient function.

BIOTIN

In addition to dietary change and exercise, biotin can be beneficial. Biotin, or vitamin H as it is often called, has been shown to stimulate production of CYP1B1 thereby elevating its level. Biotin has also been shown to inhibit NFkB, a transcriptional factor that is important in tumour survival. Relatively small amounts of biotin accomplish this.

Biotin is a non-selective inducer of enzymes. If one is receiving chemotherapy biotin would not be recommended because this induction of enzymes would result in a decrease in the effectiveness of the chemotherapy due to its metabolism by the enzymes induced by biotin.

If one has switched to a diet high in organic fruits, vegetables and whole foods one is likely getting a sufficient amount of biotin in one's diet.

The following fruits and vegetables are sources of biotin:

apple	broad beans	raspberry
artichoke (globe)	cauliflower	rhubarb
avocado	chard	strawberry
banana	grapefruit	tomato
black & red currant	peas	watermelon

(This list is illustrative rather than exhaustive.)

If biotin supplements are used 1mg (1000ug) per day would be sufficient. It would not be productive to take more than this amount per day.

MAGNESIUM AND NIACIN (VITAMIN B3)

A further benefit comes from niacin, or nicotinamide and magnesium. Niacin and magnesium stimulate the salvestrol activation reaction. This is accomplished through achieving the Recommended Dietary Allowance (RDA) for each. Research has indicated that the activity of CYP1B1 is reduced by 50% when adequate levels of magnesium are not present.

To achieve the appropriate level of niacin or nicotinamide it is a good idea to obtain this through taking a medium strength, B complex, vitamin product as this will avoid disequilibrium of other B vitamins in the body. Once again if one has made the change to a diet rich in fruits, vegetables and whole foods one is very likely to be achieving these levels through one's diet.

The following fruits and vegetables are sources of magnesium:

artichoke (globe)	chard	okra
avocado	figs	peas
banana	kale	pumpkin
beans	lettuce	savoy
broccoli	mushrooms	spinach

(This list is illustrative rather than exhaustive.)

The following fruits and vegetables are sources of niacin:

asparagus	dates	peach
avocado	figs	potato with skin
broccoli	kale	rhubarb
carrot	lettuce	spinach
chard	mango	sweet potato
corn	mushrooms	tomato

(This list is illustrative rather than exhaustive.)

IRON

CYP1B1, like other CYP enzymes, utilises iron, at its core, to oxidise various compounds that enter the body. This is the way in which CYP1B1 is able to metabolise salvestrols into the metabolites that induce cell death in the diseased cell. Cancer sufferers are often anaemic, a situation that interferes with the biogenesis of rescue enzymes like CYP1B1. Given this it is important that the Recommended Dietary Allowance (RDA) for iron is achieved either through the diet or supplementation. Those that are anaemic should discuss their iron requirements with their physician.

In our diets iron comes in two forms: iron; and heme iron. Heme iron is readily absorbed where iron is not. Sources of heme iron are meat, poultry, fish and shellfish. Sources of iron are fruits, vegetables, herbs and seeds. When iron is obtained from vegetarian sources it is important to also take vitamin C from dietary sources during the same meal to aid in the absorption of the iron. Plants are less efficient sources of iron than animal foods.

The following are sources of heme iron:

beef	halibut	tuna
chicken liver	oyster	turkey
clam	pork	
crab	shrimp	

(This list is illustrative rather than exhaustive.)

The following fruits, vegetables and herbs are sources of iron:

apricot	grape	pumpkin
artichoke	paprika	rosemary
black currant	peach	spinach
cabbage	peas	thyme

cinnamon	plum	watercress
figs	potato	

(This list is illustrative rather than exhaustive.)

VITAMIN C

Dietary sources of vitamin C should be included to aid in the absorption of plant sources of iron. Vitamin C also stimulates the immune system to assist the body in getting rid of cell debris resulting from apoptosis. A further benefit of Vitamin C comes from it serving as a sacrificial antioxidant to prevent degradation of salvestrols in the body. Orthomolecular physicians have used Vitamin C as part of their treatment regime for cancer patients for many, many years (*Fuller F, 2011*).

The following fruits, vegetables and herbs are sources of vitamin C:

black currant	loganberry	red currant
broccoli	orange	rose hip
brussels sprout	papaya	strawberry
guava	parsley	wolfberry
kiwifruit	plum	
lemon	red pepper	

(This list is illustrative rather than exhaustive.)

If vitamin C supplements are used 1gram 3 times a day would be sufficient. Consult a physician if you want to take more. Cofactor summary:

COFACTOR:	DAILY DOSE:
Biotin	1mg
Magnesium	RDA
Niacin (vitamin B3)	RDA
Iron	RDA
Vitamin C	1 – 3g

A FEW VERY GOOD FOODS

There are a number of foods that not only provide salvestrols, they also provide a variety of the important cofactors: biotin, magnesium, niacin, iron and vitamin C.

Incorporation of foods that will provide both salvestrols and cofactors will assist in achieving the full benefit of the salvestrols. Of course this will work out to maximum advantage if these foods are obtained from organic sources. Examples of such foods are provided in each of three categories: Fruits; Herbs; and vegetables below.

Salvestrol rich fruit:	Cofactors present:				
black currants:	biotin			iron	vitamin C
figs:		magnesium	niacin	iron	
raspberries:	biotin	magnesium			vitamin C

Salvestrol rich herb:	Cofactors present:				
basil:		magnesium	niacin	iron	vitamin C
mint:		magnesium	niacin	iron	vitamin C
parsley:		magnesium	niacin	iron	vitamin C

Salvestrol rich vegetable:	Cofactors present:				
avocado:	biotin	magnesium	niacin	iron	vitamin C
chard:	biotin	magnesium	niacin	iron	vitamin C
garden peas:	biotin	magnesium	niacin	iron	vitamin C
green beans:	biotin	magnesium	niacin	iron	vitamin C

After looking over these three lists of particularly beneficial foods one wonders how to conveniently take advantage of them. Here is a suggestion: incorporate them into a wrap.

Chop avocado, chard, garden peas, green beans, fresh basil and fresh parsley.

Mix two tablespoons of organic, stone ground olive oil, crushed raspberries, crushed blackcurrants and black pepper to make a salad dressing.

Mix the dressing in with the chopped vegetables and herbs. Add to the wrap. Roll up the wrap and serve!

Assuming organic ingredients, this wrap will deliver salvestrols, biotin, magnesium, niacin, iron and vitamin C all in one convenient and easy to prepare snack.

8.

THE FOOD BASIS OF THE SALVESTROL CONCEPT

Salvestrols are *"The most significant breakthrough in nutrition since the discovery of vitamins."*

❖ DAN BURKE, PH.D.

With the Salvestrol Concept it is important to remember that it is a food-based rescue mechanism. This may well be the most magnificent feature of these discoveries. We tend to forget the value of our food and view it simply as fuel or a pleasant diversion while enjoying the company of family and friends. The Salvestrol Concept helps us remember the importance of our food and the importance of quality food. It is food that sustains our life and as the Salvestrol Concept so elegantly illustrates food can help us to sustain and regain good health.

CYP1B1 metabolises salvestrols that are found in our food (fruits; vegetables; and herbs) to bring about the destruction of diseased cells. In this regard the Salvestrol Concept is not reliant on our finding some special berry, fruit, vegetable or root in some far off land.

HISTORIC INTAKE OF SALVESTROLS

This rescue mechanism first developed in mammals around 150 million years ago and covers the globe. Salvestrol rich foods are indigenous to each continent. We need not worry that only the berries common to the foothills of the Himalayas, or the Amazon jungle or the temperate rain forest of Haida Gwaii will contain the ingredients of this salvestrol rescue mechanism. We will find the salvestrols in our back garden regardless of where we live.

The difficulty, as we have discussed, is the depletion of salvestrols in the modern diet. Research indicates that the diet, up to Victorian times would include approximately 12mg of salvestrols on a daily basis. By contrast the modern diet would supply only 2mg of salvestrols daily.

THE SALVESTROL POINT SYSTEM

To translate this research into practical guidance in obtaining adequate levels of salvestrols, the researchers at Nature's Defence have formulated a points system and set of recipes.

As mentioned earlier it is selectivity that is the most desirable feature of an anticancer agent, that is, an agent that targets cancer cells while leaving healthy tissue unharmed. The more selective the anticancer agent the more potent and useful it is. Each salvestrol differs in its selectivity. What this means is that you would need a different amount, in terms of milligrams of salvestrol, for each salvestrol to have the same effect. For example, 1mg of S55 would be equal to 2,300mg of S40.

Our diet never delivers a single nutrient – it delivers a multitude of nutrients, salvestrols included. This, of course, is very beneficial. We can realise both the nutrients we need, such as a salvestrols, along with beneficial cofactors and other nutrients that support good health.

Given this, measuring salvestrol content in milligrams, as is typical with pharmaceuticals, is not appropriate. In order to take into account the differences in selectivity of the various salvestrols and to include any of the salvestrols that could occur in a food a point scheme was devised to standardise the overall salvestrol level.

The point system takes the dietary intake of the Victorian diet as the minimum recommended daily intake. The 12mg salvestrol component of the Victorian diet has been assigned 100 salvestrol points and this 100 salvestrol points represents the minimum that should be achieved on a daily basis to maintain wellbeing. The 2mg of salvestrols typically found in the modern diet represent 17 salvestrol points at best. An individual in good health should consume 350 salvestrol points daily for maintenance of good health. Those that are combating advanced disease would require much higher levels of salvestrols. Pharmacokinetic research indicates that after ingestion salvestrols will follow a standard pattern of relatively quickly achieving a peak concentration in the blood and then tapering off towards no concentration. Further to this the research indicates that the metabolic activity will be more productive and last longer if salvestrols are consumed, in volume, at the same time (such as during a meal) rather than in smaller amounts throughout the day.

Taking one's daily allotment of salvestrol points throughout the day fits with the historic, dietary intake of salvestrols, that is, via the daily meals and snacks, and helps to maintain a more consistent level of salvestrols in the blood throughout the day. This leaves the night as a time for the body to rid itself of cells that have been killed off during the day.

The 'Salvestrol Richest Recipes', that stemmed from analysis of over 8000 recipes, outlines the number of salvestrol points that would be obtained from a typical serving of each recipe. The recipe book assumes the use of non-organic fruits, vegetables and herbs as these are the most common. The salvestrol point assignment for a given recipe can be tripled if the ingredients are from organic sources.

RECIPES: SALVESTROL POINTS IN PRACTICE

To show you how the point system works we can consider a very simple recipe of small, wild carrots with fresh mint to accompany the main elements of an evening meal.

The carrots would be washed but not pealed, lightly boiled and served with butter, a drop of honey and garnished with fresh mint. A typical serving would be 3 carrots per person. Such a serving would provide the recipient with 5 salvestrol points. If the carrots and mint were obtained from organic sources each recipient would receive 15 salvestrol points from this element of the meal.

By combining salvestrol rich elements of each meal along with salvestrol rich snacks one can achieve 100 salvestrol points each day. However, one will find it dramatically easier to achieve the 100 salvestrol points with an organic diet.

Don't worry about consuming more than 100 salvestrol points in a day. Salvestrols are part of our food supply and exceeding 100 salvestrol points will be perfectly safe.

To reach the 100 salvestrol points on a daily basis one may need to significantly increase fruit, vegetable and herb consumption. Extrapolating from the carrot recipe we can see that one would have to eat 60 non-organically grown carrots, prepared according to this recipe, to achieve 100 salvestrol points. These points would be realised by only 20 organically grown carrots prepared according to this recipe. Of course, no one is going to consume this many carrots in a day. If we look at this illustration from the viewpoint of units of fruit and vegetables, rather than focusing on the carrots alone, we can see that an increase in our fruit and vegetable consumption may be necessary, especially if we are using non-organically grown produce. To illustrate this point a further selection of Salvestrol Rich Recipes are found in Appendix 4.

Salvestrol recipes along with their points per serving are available from Nature's Defence.

9.

CAUSE FOR OPTIMISM

The art of medicine consists of amusing the
patient while Nature cures the disease.

❖ VOLTAIRE

Within the context of the Salvestrol Concept there are
a number of interesting or special situations and we will
briefly touch on three of them here. In particular, we will
discuss a couple of situations where the prognosis for patients utilising conventional approaches is not particularly
good.

OVARIAN CANCER

The first situation is ovarian cancer. Ovarian cancer and
its metastases have been shown to produce the CYP1B1
enzyme in particular abundance – up to six times the levels found in other cancers (*McFadyen MCE, et al., 2001*).
It stands to reason that the more CYP1B1 enzyme that

is present, the greater the chance that any salvestrols in an ovarian cancer sufferer's system will become activated and so bring about the death of the cancer cells. This is of course very good news for those who are suffering from ovarian cancer. This also argues for a diet rich in organic fruits, vegetables and hence salvestrols for people suffering from ovarian cancer.

MESOTHELIOMA

CYP1B1 has been found to be present in the malignant cells of 98% of mesothelioma cases studied, and in abundance, much as is seen in ovarian cancers. Again, it stands to reason that this abundance of CYP1B1 will facilitate cell death if sufficient levels of salvestrols are present in the bodies of mesothelioma sufferers. Given the poor prognosis for mesothelioma through conventional therapy, it might be prudent for sufferers to switch to a diet high in salvestrols.

PETS

The CYP1B1 enzyme, our rescue enzyme, as Professor Potter prefers, is expressed in other animals besides humans. A variety of fish, eel, seal, dolphin and frog, along with fruit flies, mice, rats, cows and dogs, all express the CYP1B1 enzyme or at a minimum an enzyme that is very similar. Given this, those that have seen their fruit flies dying of cancer can safely conclude that their fruit was not organic!

The dog lovers among us will be quick to recognise the importance of CYP1B1 for their pets. Many a family pet has been lost to cancer and if CYP1B1 can serve as a rescue enzyme for humans through its metabolism of salvestrols then perhaps it could serve a similar role in animals. We have all noticed that dogs will eat vegetative matter when they appear to be sick. Perhaps this is an instinctive response that enables them to capitalise on the health benefits afforded by the Salvestrol Concept.

The faster metabolism of dogs enables them to process higher levels of salvestrols more effectively than humans. Of course given the huge variability in size of dogs one would want to take the weight of the dog into consideration. As with humans it would be best to provide salvestrols with the dog's meals.

OTHER DISEASES

The salvestrol concept can be viewed as highlighting one of the bodies rescue mechanisms for killing off cells that need to be killed off. Since the lead researchers are cancer researchers the focus of their investigations has been cancer. However, there are many cells that need to be killed off and removed and there is some evidence that this mechanism is somewhat broader in scope than cancer.

While investigating diseased tissue for the presence of CYP1B1 the research team discovered that this unique enzyme is also expressed in ulcerative colitis. The significance of this is that these cells should also be killed off through the metabolism of salvestrols. A sufferer of ulcerative colitis may well gain relief from either a diet rich in organic fruits and vegetables or through salvestrol supplementation.

Autoimmune disorders are another area where increasing the level of daily salvestrol consumption appears to result in a decrease in inflammation and benefit to the individual. Autoimmune disorders are on the increase. Immune cells are supposed to die off once they have done the job that they were generated to do. In certain autoimmune disorders there is a build up of mature immune cells that, rather than dying off, continue operating, causing damage to healthy tissue. One can readily see that if the diet is deficient in salvestrols inflammation will prevail and certain autoimmune disorders, such as arthritis, will progress.

You may recall from our earlier discussion of resveratrol that the initial interest in resveratrol came from investigations of its impact on cardiovascular health. Since the newer salvestrols have been discovered there is preliminary evidence that the lipophilic salvestrol, S31G, can lower blood pressure. Further work is still needed to understand this effect more fully.

Finally, it is worth repeating that salvestrols will perform the same anti-fungal function in humans that they perform in plants. This is not to say that a salvestrol will combat any fungal infection as the salvestrols tend to be pathogen specific. However, a diet rich in a variety of organic fruits and vegetables should provide an array of salvestrols that will assist with many of the fungal infections that people typically suffer from such as Candida, athlete's foot, etc.

Although the focus of this research team is cancer these additional findings indicate that salvestrols can be of broad health benefit. Over time one anticipates that a fuller understanding of the mechanisms of cell death in other diseases and disorders will be brought to light. In the interim one will not go too far wrong by increasing one's organic fruit and vegetable consumption.

10.
LATEST DEVELOPMENTS

The best way to have a good idea is to have a
lot of ideas.

❖ LINUS PAULING

Nature's Defence is conducting a very active program of
research aimed at expanding their knowledge of salvestrols, the food sources of salvestrols, and the enzymes that
activate them, such as CYP1B1. As this understanding
of all the nuances involved in the Salvestrol Concept increases Nature's Defence will gain the insights necessary
to increase the utility of salvestrols, whether obtained from
diet, supplements or both, and cancer sufferers will be the
benefactors of this increased understanding.

SUSPECTED SYNERGY BETWEEN SALVESTROLS

S40 and S31G were the original salvestrols found in
salvestrol supplements. The central difference between

these two salvestrols is that S40 is hydrophilic while S31G is lipophilic. That is, S31G can diffuse through tissue very readily enabling it to reach throughout the body with ease. S40 is transported through the body via the circulatory system.

Recent observations have led researchers at Nature's Defence to suspect that there is a synergistic relationship between S40 and S31G and indeed between all of the salvestrols, resulting in greater activation and effectiveness than realised with either in isolation from the other. In addition, each unique salvestrol has its own unique nutritional benefits aside from the benefits derived from its metabolism by CYP1B1. Given that salvestrols are typically obtained from food we would consume more than one salvestrol during a meal along with a variety of salvestrol cofactors. This suspected synergy follows the typical ingestion pattern for salvestrols.

THE 5 SERIES OF SALVESTROLS

S55 is a member of a new generation of salvestrols that was recently found. As we have seen the potency of anticancer agents is measured in terms of their selectivity. That is, their ability to kill cancer cells without harming healthy tissue. S55 has selectivity equal to or greater than that achieved by the Stilserene prodrug that Professor Potter developed to target CYP1B1. This is an extremely powerful, targeted, food-based compound. The 5 series of salvestrols holds great promise and remains the focus of considerable research.

Discovery of the 5 series of salvestrols underscores the ongoing commitment to research found at Nature's

Defence. The search for more interesting salvestrols is an ongoing process.

NEW PRODUCT DEVELOPMENT

With the discovery of a new and highly powerful new generation of salvestrols, researchers at Nature's Defence are working on deepening their understanding of these compounds so that ultimately they can be incorporated into new products.

The discovery of the salvestrol concept has pointed out that the approach taken with salvestrols is a fruitful approach to apply to other diseases as well as to more focused approaches to specific cancers. As time and resources permit research will be expanded to include these new directions. Every effort will be made to combine disease pathway understanding with food screening to bring further beneficial classes of phytonutrients to light.

CASE STUDIES

Over the past few years the research team has had occasion to follow the progress of individuals using salvestrols as part of their approach to overcoming their cancer. In 2007 five individuals agreed to participate in case studies. The cancers that these individuals were diagnosed as having included: stage 2-3 squamous-cell carcinoma of the lung; stage 4 melanoma; prostate cancer; aggressive, stage 3 breast cancer; and bladder cancer. Each of these individuals had a complete recovery from their cancer (Schaefer B, 2007). In 2010 an additional six individuals agreed to participate in case studies. The cancers that these individuals were diagnosed as having included: stage 3 breast cancer; stage 2 liver cancer; colon cancer; a recurrent prostate cancer; a further prostate cancer with a Gleason score of 6 (3+3); and a stage 3 B Hodgkin's lymphoma. Again all six individuals had a complete recovery from their cancer (Schaefer B, 2010).

The monitoring of individuals, through their case study participation, has lead us to belief that those individuals with the best responses are those that embrace dietary and lifestyle change in concert with their use of salvestrols. It would appear that a move towards a more organic diet with a greater emphasis on fruit and vegetable consumption along with at least a modest exercise program will go a long way to realising benefit from salvestrols.

These case studies have also brought to light the fact that certain individuals respond exceptionally quickly to salvestrols. In addition, certain individuals respond very favourably to low doses of salvestrol. Although these individuals represent a minority of those that benefit from salvestrols they raise important questions for further research. What is it about these individuals that results in either the rapid response or the low dose response? Are they more efficient at absorbing salvestrols? Are they more efficient at metabolising salvestrols? Further research will hopefully shed some light on these questions.

At present a follow up study is underway to track the progress of these 11 individuals. Upon completion of this study the results will be made available through publication. Further to this a variety of individuals are currently participating in new case studies. Upon completion we will be publishing new cases representing stage 1 breast cancer, squamous cell carcinoma of the anus, ovarian cancer, benign prostatic hyperplasia, and chronic lymphocytic leukaemia. Case studies represent an important component of the overall research effort and will constitute an ongoing area of research investigation.

PRACTITIONER TRAINING

Many practitioners have expressed an interest in receiving training in the various aspects of salvestrols and their use. In response to this demand Nature's Defence has developed a Practitioner Training Program to address this need.

The training program consists of various modules with a question and answer session at the end of each module. Practitioners are encouraged to discuss the research presented. The various modules enable the participants to:

- ❖ Recognise applications for Salvestrols
- ❖ Use Salvestrols successfully for your patients' health
- ❖ Identify factors that influence the effectiveness of Salvestrols
- ❖ Recommend a diet to complement Salvestrol use
- ❖ Make considered decisions about the use of Salvestrols
- ❖ Explore with colleagues the potential use of Salvestrols
- ❖ Start to understand the underlying science of Salvestrols
- ❖ Ask informed questions about Salvestrols

Successful completion of the courses will result in a certificate stating that the recipient is suitably qualified to offer advice on salvestrols. Certificate holders will also be published on the relevant salvestrol website so that prospective customers can locate them easily.

11.
TOOLS FOR EARLY CANCER DETECTION

Whether you think you can, or you think you can't – you're right.

❖ HENRY FORD

Over the years the research team has held many discussions that revolved around the need for better clinical tools in cancer research. In 2007 we took the decision to tackle this need and formed a new company called CARE Biotechnologies Inc., to carry out research aimed at realising such tools. Researchers at CARE Biotechnologies are working on the development of two separate blood tests for the early detection of cancer, the monitoring of disease progression, the individualisation of treatment and the monitoring of individuals in remission.

THE NEED FOR NEW CLINICAL TOOLS

The difficulty with existing clinical tools is twofold. Current technology can only detect cancer once the cancer has grown to between 10^8 and 10^9 cells (if you look at the nail on your little finger, half that size is between 10^8 and 10^9 cells – roughly the size of a pea) – once cancer reaches 10^{12} cells (about a litre of cells) you're dead. By the time modern technology can tell you that you have this disease the disease has silently grown through about 75% of its life. (Dan Burke wrote an excellent article of this topic: *Burke, MD, 2009*).

The other side of the problem is that once you are told that you have this disease there are really poor tools, for most of the cancers, for monitoring disease progression and treatment efficacy as well as the detection of disease recurrence.

In Figure 3 we can see the implications of the silent growth of cancer. The area in gray represents the undetected growth of the cancer.

This has implications for people that start to think about cancer prevention. They, of course, assume that they are free of the disease. They may consult a physician and take advice on cancer prevention. But this advice is also likely to assume that they are free of the disease, however, they may lie anywhere on that curve below the level of detection. If they are already up that curve preventive doses are going to slow the rate of cancer growth but not keep the cancer from breaking through into the detectable range.

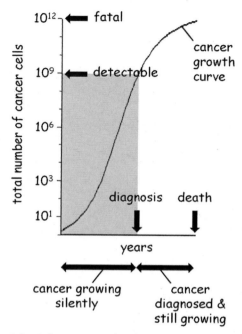

Figure 3. The Silent Growth of Cancer. Reprinted with the kind permission of Prof. Dan Burke.

The silent growth of cancer figure also has implications for people that have journeyed through this disease to the point that their physician has told them that they are 'all clear'. This statement may simply mean that their disease is again below the level of detection. They may, in fact, be clear of this disease have no more cancer cells in their body than any healthy person. However, the 'all clear' could also mean that the attending physician simply could no longer detect cancer cells in a situation where there is an abundance of cancer cells present just below technology's level of detection, that is, within the silent growth of cancer area. This is a very probable scenario for those individuals that are given the 'all clear' and are then re-diagnosed within the next couple of years. Consideration of the silent growth of cancer would strongly suggest that anyone given the 'all clear' carry on with beneficial dietary and lifestyle changes, including incorporating more salvestrols in their diet, to ensure that the level of resident cancer cells diminishes well below the level of detection.

All in all this amounts to a pretty miserable picture.

Wouldn't it be great if we had a simple blood test that could be used to screen for any of the cancers, with a sensitivity that could pick up the presence of the disease long before it has reached 10^8 and 10^9 cells? Think about how much easier it would be to assist these people back to good health - and wouldn't it be nice if a simple blood test could be used to monitor any of the cancers with a level of accuracy that would readily tell if a treatment is working or not and whether a dose is high enough? A blood test that is as applicable and accurate with pancreatic cancer as it is with breast cancer – a blood test that is as applicable and accurate with adrenal cancer as it is with prostate cancer. Tools such as these could make life a lot easier for clinicians and patients alike.

DEVELOPMENT OF CLINICAL TOOLS FOR EARLY CANCER DETECTION AND MONITORING

The need for new clinical tools is obvious. One of the enormous implications of the prior work of Professors Potter and Burke is that it sets the stage for the realisation of blood tests such as those that I just described.

We started to look at what we had to work with. We had great expertise on CYP enzymes and we had great expertise on secondary plant metabolites and their metabolism by CYP enzymes. Specifically, we had CYP1B1, a universal cancer marker and salvestrols, natural prodrugs, which in this context amounts to things to look for in bodily fluids. Given the salvestrol – CYP1B1 mechanism there should be things that we could look for that would tell us about the presence and state of this disease. Basically we could use our understanding of this metabolic relationship to report back to us on the disease itself.

We took the decision to utilise this knowhow and develop clinical tools for the early detection of all cancers, and treatment efficacy – no small challenge! To this end one thing that we have learned so far on this project is that it is a really good idea to have people on your research team that don't know that it can't be done!

In considering the problem we decided that we had one of two directions to take. The obvious first route was to develop a method for detecting and measuring the presence of CYP1B1 itself. Since CYP1B1 is an intrinsic component of cancer cells if we could detect and measure it in blood or urine we would have a direct measure of the disease itself. The second, and much less obvious approach was to develop a method for detecting and measuring the metabolic output of CYP1B1. If we could find a strong metabolic output of CYP1B1, detect and measure it we would have another direct measure of this disease. So we decided to pursue both – two universal tests for cancer.

PROTEOMIC APPROACH:

In pursuing the detection and measurement of CYP1B1 itself we knew that the job would be made much easier if we had an antibody – something to help us isolate CYP1B1 from everything else found in blood. Specifically we wanted an antibody to an amino acid string that was 100% specific to CYP1B1, covering the wild form and the major polymorphs and not found in any bacteria. We also wanted one that didn't have major cleavage sites (sites where the string could be digested and broken) running through the middle of it. These criteria ruled out all of the antibodies that are currently available for CYP1B1. We performed an exhaustive search and identified a set of peptides that met our criteria and embarked on raising antibodies.

CYP1B1 is a very difficult enzyme to raise antibodies for that have a strong affinity for the peptide of interest because CYP1B1 is present in so many life forms in identical form or near identical form to that found in humans. However, we did manage to raise an antibody to a specific CYP1B1 peptide and worked on affinity enhancement until we had something useable.

Our first notion was to see if we could detect and measure CYP1B1 in human tumour samples. Seemed like a good idea at the time – where else are we going to find CYP1B1 in abundance?

We spent about a year working on sample preparation methods and testing samples using some of the world's most sophisticated mass spectrometry equipment. We spiked the tumour matrix with CYP1B1 from recombinant sources and managed to recover the recombinant material but never managed to detect the native CYP1B1. This caused us some considerable concern because the wisdom of the day dictated that if we couldn't manage to detect and measure CYP1B1 in tumour samples, where it would be plentiful, we would never be able to detect and measure it in blood or urine. Given that we were able to detect and measure the recombinant CYP from the tumour matrix we knew that we had a sample preparation and extraction problem – we were either not freeing the enzyme from the surrounding material or we were destroying the enzyme with our preparation method.

In light of this we decided to abandon our search for CYP1B1 in tissue and focus on detecting it in blood. This decision flew in the face of conventional wisdom but our thought was that if we were ever going to have a viable diagnostic and monitoring tool it had to work on blood or urine samples so if we were going to pound our heads against a wall it might as well be the wall we needed to climb. It isn't really as crazy as it initially sounds – even though everyone told us that we were crazy. When working with blood you don't need some of the sample prep steps that you would use with tissue because you don't have as much intact material to deal with – you are already working with fragments.

So we embarked on trying to find our CYP1B1 peptide in blood. We ended up with the same results as we found for tissue! We spiked recombinant CYP1B1 into blood and managed to recover it but were unable to recover native CYP1B1 amidst a chorus of 'I told you so' until one member of the team came up with the bright idea of starting with more blood! We increased the initial sample size and detected and measured our native peptide.

PROTEOMIC RESULTS

The naturally present CYP1B1 peptide was successfully detected using antibody-affinity capture in both 20 µl and 200 µl digests of cancer patient plasma. The amount of natural CYP1B1 in this sample was estimated to be ~200 amol/µl of plasma. The result was then replicated with 5 additional samples:

Sample	Amount of CYP1B1 (amol/µl of plasma)
1	12.5
2	2.0
3	9.4
4	9.2
5	4.9

Lower levels of peptide were found in these samples with the amount of natural CYP1B1 ranging from 2 to 12.5 amol/µl of plasma (*Schaefer B, 2010*).

Further improvements were made to our sample preparation methods and more extensive testing began with clinical samples from individuals suffering from colorectal cancer, ovarian cancer and lung cancer. We were able to detect our peptide, and hence CYP1B1 in all these cancers. Further to this we were able to detect CYP1B1 in a proteomic standard – a sample of plasma that represents plasma, obtained from a large array of healthy individuals, that has had specific quantities of known blood components added to it for the purpose of calibrating analytical instruments such as mass spectrometers. The detection of CYP1B1 in a proteomic standard serves as our measure of baseline levels found in healthy individuals until further testing is accomplished. The level found in the proteomic standard was as minute as one would expect given that healthy individuals have very few cancer cells on any given day.

With the samples obtained from lung cancer patients the levels of CYP1B1 measured were between 92 and 6291 times the background level in a proteomic standard and represented a good match to level of disease progression.

From this data we returned to the silent growth of cancer figure and made some calculations to estimate where this data would set a new detection limit. In figure 4 we see that by applying this proteomic cancer test we estimate that we would be able to detect lung cancer approximately 5.7 years earlier than existing technology. Frankly put, in the life cycle of lung cancer, detection of the cancer 5.7 years earlier than it is currently being detected is the difference between red roses and white roses, the difference between laughter and tears - life where death is probable.

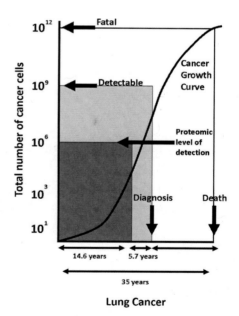

Figure 4. New limit of detection for lung cancer.

PROTEOMIC SUMMARY

At this point we have a sample preparation method and an antibody (an assay) that is able to directly detect and measure cancer though detection of CYP1B1 in plasma. When we find our peptide in your blood with this assay you have cancer – there are no false positives – you have cancer.

We have been working on research machines but we have now identified a mass spectrometer that is designed for use in clinical laboratories and we believe that this machine will enable us to deliver this assay for routine use in clinical laboratories.

We now have a variety of method enhancement experiments, stability experiments, validation experiments and method transfer experiments to conduct but at least at this point we know it is present in the blood, we can find it and we can measure it. One of the strengths of this approach is that it will be simple and convenient for the person getting tested. Simply put out your arm for a sample collection like any other blood test. What I also like about this approach is that it is a direct detection and measurement of the cancer itself and it is as applicable to pancreatic cancer as it is to breast cancer – it is applicable to all the cancers. Another strength of this test is that it is operating at an exceptionally high level of sensitivity and we have good reason to believe that we can increase the level of sensitivity from here.

METABOLITE APPROACH

We know the various substrates of CYP1B1, that is, we know what it metabolizes and in particular we know a lot about the salvestrols that it metabolizes. So what happens when we ingest salvestrols?

In our food salvestrols come in two forms: as a glycoside and as an aglycone – in food about 80% as glycosides and 20% aglycones – in capsules 100% aglycones. When we ingest the glycoside the plant sugar is cleaved off and replaced with a human sugar. When we ingest the aglycone a human sugar is attached. This of course assumes that everything is working properly to perform this function. The new glycoside is then transported and upon reaching cancer cells the human sugar is cleaved off leaving the aglycone at the cancer site. This step is performed by Beta Glucoronidase. The aglycone then binds with CYP1B1 and is metabolized. The metabolite induces apoptosis spilling the contents of the cancer cell, including CYP1B1 peptides and metabolites into the surrounding space. What all this means for blood test development is that the interaction of CYP1B1 and salvestrols provides us with a variety of measurable aspects of this process that can provide us with insights into the presence of disease as certain of these aspects can only be present if the disease is present and metabolism has taken place.

What we did initially is go through our list of salvestrols looking for metabolites that were abundantly produced through CYP1B1 metabolism and not found in a typical diet. From a candidate list one metabolite was chosen.

We looked to see if we could find the aglycone in blood and urine – initially used predicted structures and then using synthesized standards we were able to reliably detect and measure the aglycone in both blood and urine. We then performed a pharmacokinetic study using healthy volunteers to determine when salvestrols reach peak concentration in the blood – three hours after ingestion. We identified the aglycone spike resulting from salvestrol using hplc (high performance liquid chromatography, a standard analytical technique for the separation of compounds in a complex mixture). Prior to hplc analysis the samples were prepared and Beta Glucuronidase was used to remove the sugar from the glycoside, thereby pooling the glycoside and aglycone into a single signal.

Following this we decided to take a look and see if we could find a difference between healthy volunteers and those with advanced cancers. We administered 1 gram of a specific salvestrol to each individual, waited 3 hours and drew their blood. We also had each individual do a 24 hour urine collection. As expected, with healthy volunteers we found no metabolite – we simply recovered the substrate (the salvestrol) in blood and urine. With diseased volunteers the situation was very different. We found a very clear spike on the hplc where we predicted that the metabolite should come off the column. Some of these individuals had really very advanced disease and with these individuals we found absolutely no aglycone and no glycoside – just metabolite. When we analysed their urine we also found no aglycone. The entire gram of substrate seemed to have been used up. With other cancer patients we found small amounts of aglycone along with large metabolite spikes. What this tells us is that the ratio of metabolite to aglycone may be of much greater clinical value than the metabolite alone – time will tell. We performed these tests with individuals representing a fairly broad array of common cancers: breast, stomach, kidney, prostate, etc., and an array of stages of cancer but skewed towards more advanced cancers. Metabolite spikes were found for all as one would expect given that we are looking at the metabolic output of a universal cancer marker.

METABOLITE SUMMARY

So at this point we have a sample preparation method that allows us to detect the aglycone and the metabolite in blood or urine using hplc. We find clear separations between the outputs obtained from healthy volunteers as compared to diseased volunteers. Like the proteomic approach when we find this metabolite in your blood you have cancer.

A magnificent strength of this approach is that it uses natural products as diagnostics. We are getting the metabolism of a natural product to report on the presence and state of disease. Another nice feature of this approach is that we can build the signal by the amount of substrate that we administer. A further strength of this approach is that it not only tells us that CYP1B1 is present, that is that cancer is present, it can tell us that the enzyme is functioning properly.

We have been drawing blood at 3 hours, the time of peak concentration for the substrate. We are about to embark on a pharmacokinetic study to determine peak concentration of the metabolite. Once we are able to draw blood coincident with peak concentration of the metabolite we will be able to pick up the presence of cancer much earlier as this will give us the maximum signal for the amount of salvestrol administered. Like the proteomic test the metabolite test is universally applicable.

SO WHERE ARE WE?

A present we have two different assays for detecting and measuring the presence and amount of cancer. Both operate independent of any apriori notions about type of cancer that may be present.

The huge strength of these approaches is that they can be used with all cancers – they are two universal cancer tests that can ultimately be used for diagnosis and monitoring across all of the cancers. The downside of this is that we will need to validate both approaches on each and every cancer which means that there is a great deal of validation work in front of us.

Up 'till now everyone on the team has had their pet blood test – either the metabolite test or the proteomic test. However, from the onset there have been good arguments for seeing both of these approaches through to completion because they provide differing set of strengths and weaknesses. When we combine them we can potentially provide much more clinical assistance that we could with results from either one.

A POSSIBLE SCENARIO USING BOTH TESTS

For example, let's say that we have two 36 year old females, very similar in family history, medical history, etc., and both have a 2 cm cancerous lump in one of their breasts. Their physician decides to run the metabolite test. With one of the women a large metabolite spike is found with no aglycone and no glycoside. With the other woman we find a medium sized spike of metabolite and small spikes of aglycone and glycoside. What is going on? With just the metabolite test we might conclude that woman number 1 has fully functioning CYP1B1 that is making full use of the substrate while woman number 2 may have competing substrates in her body that are inhibiting the functioning of CYP1B1 – for example she may have been using some household paints that contain chemical anti-fungal agents or perhaps she had the furnace duct work recently cleaned and the cleaners used chemical anti-fungal agents to retard any fungal build up or perhaps she takes daily walks along the perimeter of a golf course that uses a great deal of anti-fungal spraying. We may also conclude that woman number 1 may have an additional undetected tumour mass. If we now run the proteomic test we can help to determine what in fact is going on for these two women. Let's say that we run the proteomic test and find a larger spike of peptide for woman number 1 than woman number 2. This result would tell us that there may be no difference at all between the functioning of CYP1B1 for these two women but rather confirm that woman number 1 has another, undetected tumour mass and this is accounting for the higher results. The attending clinician can then embark on a search for the whereabouts of this second tumour mass.

WHERE DO WE WANT TO GET TO?

The research and development to date has given us confidence that a simple blood or urine test will be delivered for early cancer detection. We are confident that a cost effective and minimally invasive means of monitoring each of the cancers will be realised. It is the hope of this research team that test sensitivity will be such that through the use of these tests clinicians will be able to rapidly determine whether or not a treatment is working or whether or not the dose of a treatment has been appropriate. This could significantly improve a clinician's ability to tailor the treatment regime to the needs of the patient.

Finally, the researcher team is confident that a minimally invasive means of monitoring those individuals that are in remission will be realised. Monitoring of remission could amount to nothing more than an additional tick on a clinical laboratory requisition form upon the conclusion of a medical examination.

Along with this diagnostic development, logistical work is being carried out to determine the best way of cost-effectively delivering these tests to those that wish to use them.

12.
CONCLUSION

It takes approximately forty years for innovative
thought to be incorporated into mainstream
thought. I expect and hope that orthomolecular
medicine, within the next five to ten years,
will cease to be a speciality in medicine and
that all physicians will be using nutrition as an
essential tool in treating disease.

❖ABRAM HOFFER, M.D., PH.D

The Monks that took in our distraught friend may well
have stumbled upon the Salvestrol Concept, not from a
scientific perspective, but rather from common sense and
observation.

The Monks likely enjoy good health and longevity
from their vegetarian diets with little, if any, incidence of
cancer. We can be fairly certain that they are not spend-
ing their money on agrochemicals in the production of
their foods. Given the climatic conditions in which they
live there is likely an abundance of fresh fruit available to

them year round affording them the luxury of picking the fruit after it has ripened on the tree. As we have seen these factors contribute to fruits with high levels of salvestrols.

By providing this young man with a diet consisting of abundant fruits and unfiltered fruit juices they would have supplied him with therapeutic levels of salvestrols. As the Salvestrol Concept outlines, the salvestrols would have entered his blood stream and been delivered to the cancer cells. Upon entering the cancer cells the salvestrols would encounter the CYP1B1 enzyme and their metabolism into an anticancer agent would have taken place. The resultant metabolite would then have initiated the cascade of processes within the cancer cell that result in its death. This process continued day by day until all of the cancer had been destroyed and the dead cancer cells had been removed from his body. For our distraught friend, like the Monks that took him in, food was central to his rescue mechanism.

So where do we go from here? We know that our food is not providing the nutrition and minerals that it used to and this likely explains the amazing growth in availability and consumption of organic produce and food supplements. As Professor Harry Foster points out "The ever declining mineral content of soils, and foods grown in them, requires that the public take supplements, if only to keep their mineral intake at former levels." Given this and our new found understanding of the salvestrol concept a trip to your local organic produce supplier and health food store would be a good start.

When you pick up food to take home for your family give a moment's consideration to whether or not there was anything in the growing of this food or its processing that would have removed or diminished its food value. If yes, you may wish to look for an alternative choice. If the answer remains yes you may wish to supplement. This start may well keep you from a desperate, last minute search for a monastery!

What lies ahead? Professors Potter and Burke have provided us with an enormous step forward through the salvestrol concept but much work remains to be done. The quest for new salvestrols continues. New salvestrols with interesting and unique characteristics, selectivity and activity are continually being found.

Research continues on enzymes related to CYP1B1. Nature has likely provided a back-up mechanism to the salvestrol concept and this back-up mechanism may well be closely related to CYP1B1.

Pre-existing conditions or further disorders that arise subsequently often accompany cancer. This appears to be especially true among seniors. Given this, a large variety of anecdotal reports have been gathered that suggest that salvestrols can assist with other disease. Of particular interest here is autoimmune disorders. Many seniors afflicted with cancer also suffer from one or other autoimmune disorder. Many of these people have reported alleviation of the symptoms of their autoimmune disorders, especially arthritis, after taking salvestrols. Early work on providing a theoretical framework for understanding this phenomenon has begun. As time and resources permit, this phenomenon will be investigated to bring to light the mechanism(s) that may account for it. For the time being these reports simply argue further for a diet rich in organic fruits, vegetables and herbs.

Of considerable research interest is the population of cancer sufferers that do not respond to salvestrols or do not respond to them in a timely enough fashion. Is this due to one or other polymorphism of CYP1B1, the levels of CYP1B1 being expressed, exposure to inhibitors of CYP1B1, a combination of these factors or factors that are at present unknown? Research into illuminating a back-up rescue mechanism and the food-based compounds that it utilises is hoped to help this population to benefit from salvestrols. Recent work on the metabolism of the Salvestrol S55 shows great promise in this regard. Research indicates that the enzyme profile of very advanced cancers is different than that of less advanced cancers. S55 appears to be metabolised by CYP1B1 into a compound with anti-cancer properties as well as being metabolised by enzymes found only in advanced cancers. Further research aimed at deepening the understanding of this potential back-up mechanism will remain central areas of interest for this research team.

The salvestrol concept that resulted from the work of Professors Potter and Burke has given us a molecular level explanation of the link between diet and cancer. The current research on development of cancer diagnostics will help us to expand this concept and deepen our level of understanding. Perhaps this new understanding will usher in a new array of cancer stories - uplifting cancer stories of survival!

If you need to visit a monastery then by all means visit a monastery. If it is health and wellbeing that is on your mind then revisit the Salvestrol Concept, change your diet to include abundant, organic fruits, vegetables and herbs, and let the Monks get on with their meditation.

GLOSSARY

Abiraterone acetate	a CYP17 inhibitor, designed by Professor Potter, that is used in last line prostate cancer treatment
aglycone	the non-sugar compound that results from hydrolysis of a glycoside
antioxidant	a chemical compound that inhibits oxidation
antineoplastic drugs	anticancer drugs used to kill neoplastic cells; side effects include nausea, hair loss, and suppression of bone marrow function
apoptosis	disintegration of damaged or unwanted cells. The bodies mechanism for ridding itself of cells (programmed cell death)
carcinogenic	a substance that causes cancer
chiral	compounds having different left and right-handed forms
CYP17	a cytochrome P450 enzyme that is involved in androgen and oestrogen biosynthesis

CYP1B1	a cytochrome P450 enzyme that is intrinsic to cancer cells and not found in healthy tissue
cytochrome P450 enzyme	a superfamily of hemeproteins that are found in animals, plants, fungi and bacteria. They are best known for their drug and toxin metabolism
cytotoxic	toxic to cells, kills cells
dysplastic	evidence of abnormal growth of cells, tissue or organs (dysplasia)
EROD assay	ethoxyresorufin-O-deethylase assays - the premier method of quantifying the activity of CYP enzymes
estradiol	the predominant estrogenic hormone
glycoside	a sugar combined with a compound, predominantly from plants
hplc	high-performance liquid chromatography is an analytical technique used to separate a mixture of compounds and isolate a compound of interest
hydrophilic	molecules that have an affinity for and tendency to dissolve in water. Hydrophilic salvestrols are distributed in the body via the circulatory system
hydroxylation	the introduction of one or more hydroxyl groups (-OH) into a compound – oxidising a compound

immunohistochemical	the use of stained antibodies in the identification of specific features of cell biology
lipophilic	molecules that have an affinity for and tendency to dissolve in fats (lipids). Lipophilic salvestrols are distributed in the body via the lymphatic system and by crossing from cell to cell
mass spectrometry	an analytical technique involving mass spectrometers to identify the chemicals involved in a substance by measuring mass and charge. Mass Spectrometry is heavily used in proteomic research.
microtome	preparation of a very thin slice of tissue for microscopic examination
mutagenic	an agent such as a chemical, ultraviolet light or radioactive element that can alter DNA to cause a mutation
neoplasm	A new and abnormal growth of tissue
orthomolecular	"orthomolecular medicine describes the practice of preventing and treating disease by providing the body with optimal amounts of substances which are natural to the body." www.orthomed.org
pathogen	an agent that causes disease in another organism

pharmacokinetics	study of the processes of bodily absorption, distribution, metabolism and excretion (ADME) of compounds
phytoalexin	phytoalexins are part of the plant immune system. They are metabolites produced in response to infection by fungus or other pathogen that are inhibitory to the invading pathogen
phytochemistry	a branch of chemistry dealing with the constituents of plants and in particular medicinal plants
phytoestrogen	compounds found in plants that have similar activity in animals as oestrogen
phytonutrient	compounds found in plants that have a beneficial effect on human health that are neither vitamins and minerals
piceatannol	a hydroxylated analogue of the stilbene resveratrol that has antileukaemic activity and is also a tyrosine kinase inhibitor. Piceatannol is produced when resveratrol is metabolised by CYP1B1
polymorphism	a common mutation in DNA
polyphenol	chemicals made up of multiple phenols (C_6H_5OH) which in turn are made up of a phenyl (C_6H_5) ring bonded to a hydroxyl (OH) group
pomace	the solids that remain after grapes, olives or fruits are pressed to release the juice or oil

prodrug	a drug or natural compound that relies on enzymatic bioactivation to realise its effect – therapies that would be benign until activated by enzymatic reaction
proteomics	the study of proteins, how and when they are expressed, how they function and how the interact with one another and their involvement in metabolic pathways
resveratrol	a salvestrol and natural fungicide found in the skin of grapes, peanuts, red wine, etc., that at very low doses is metabolised by the CYP1B1 enzyme in cancer cells to produce piceatannol
S31G	a lipophilic salvestrol with a selectivity value of 22
S40	a hydrophilic salvestrol with a selectivity value of 10
S52	a lipophilic salvestrol with a selectivity value of 32
S54	a lipophilic salvestrol with a selectivity value of 1,250
S55	a lipophilic salvestrol with a selectivity value of 23,000
salvestrol	natural fungicides found in fruits, vegetables and herbs that are metabolised by the CYP1B1 enzyme in cancer cells to produce a toxin that kills the cancer cell

stilbene	hydrocarbons, C14H12, that are used in the production of dyes and synthetic estrogens
Stilserene	an anticancer agent developed by Professor Potter that is completely targeted to the CYP1B1 enzyme. It is non-toxic to healthy tissue and is metabolised into a toxin by CYP1B1 within the cancer cell
substrate	a substance or compound upon which an enzyme acts to produce a metabolite

REFERENCES IN THE POPULAR PRESS

CAHN-Pro Nutrition News and Views, Professional Edition (February 12, 2012). *Nature May Have A Helper To Fight Cancer.*

Schaefer BA. December 2012. *Gerry Potter Honoured for his Development of Abiraterone Acetone, Helping HANS.* http://www.helping-hans.org/show104a2s/Gerry_Potter_Honoured_for_his_Development_of_Abiraterone_Ace

Healy, E. June 2011. *Salvestrols and skin cancer.* CAHN-Pro Nutrition News and Views, Professional Edition, Issue 7. p 1&5.

Schaefer BA, Dooner C, Burke DM, Potter GA, Winter 2010/11 *Nutrition and Cancer: Further Case Studies Involving Salvestrol. Health Action Magazine*, 11-13.

Ware, W. October 2009. *Salvestrol update.* International Health News, Issue 201, p.5. http://www.yourhealthbase.com/ihn_october2009.pdf

Schaefer, B., Dooner, C. April 2009 *Does an Apple a Day Keep the Doctor Away?*. The Bulletin, WANP.

Wakeman, M. (March 2009) *Cancer Cell Science*. Second annual conference: Cancer Prevention and Healing. . DVD available from Health Action Network Society. http://www.hans.org/store/Cancer_Prevention

Dooner, C., Schaefer, B. Spring 2009. *An Apple a Day*. CSNN Holistic Nutrition News.

Schaefer BA, Hoon LT, Burke DM, Potter GA, Spring 2008. *Nutrition and Cancer: Salvestrol Case Studies*. Health Action Magazine, 8-9. http://www.hans.org/magazine/278/Nutrition-and-Cancer-Salvestrol-Case-Studies.

Burke, D. (March 2008) *Breakthroughs in cancer research from the UK*. First annual conference: Cancer, Natural Approaches for Prevention and Healing. . DVD available from Health Action Network Society. http://www.hans.org/store/Cancer_Prevention

Schaefer, B. Summer 2008. *Salvestrols – Linking Diet and Cancer*. CSNN Holistic Nutrition News.

Ware, W. June 2008. *Salvestrols - A new approach to cancer therapy?* International Health News, Issue 188, p. 1-3. http://www.yourhealthbase.com/archives/ihn188ww.pdf

Peskett, T. Winter 2007. *Organic Wine – A Toast to Disease Prevention.* Health Action Magazine, 27. http://www.hans.org/magazine/389/Organic-Wine

Tan, H. August/September 2007. *Can Food Really be Your Medicine?* Townsend Letter, 116-119.

Schaefer, B. April 2007. *Salvestrols – Linking Diet and Cancer.* Vitality Magazine, 90-91.

Wakeman, M. Spring 2007. *My Voyage Of Discovery Of The Remarkable World Of Salvestrols.* Health Action Magazine, http://www.hans.org/magazine/339/My-Voyage-of-Discovery-from

Schaefer, B., & Tan, H. Mar/Apr 2007. *New Developments in the Science of Salvestrols.* Vista Magazine, 54-55. www.vistamagonline.com

Tan, H. Winter 2007. *Salvestrols: Important New Developments.* Health Action Magazine, 18-19.

Fenn, C. November 2006. *Get a Taste for Salvestrols. Chris Fenn explains why some bitter fruit packs a sweet surprise.* Cycling Plus, 57.

Cox, G. October 2006. *Choices:Organic Cancer-Killers?* Candis, 70-71.

Schaefer, B. Fall 2006. *Salvestrol News.* Health Action Magazine, 30.

Hancock, M. October 2006. *Modern fruits and*

veggies in a nutritional slump. Alive Magazine, 36–37.

Schaefer, B. Summer 2006. *Salvestrols vs Cancer: The Story Continues.* Health Action Magazine, 26-27. http://www.hans.org/magazine/355/Salvestrols-vs-Cancer-The-Story-Continues

Underhill, L. July/Aug 2006. *From Red Wine to Bean Sprouts.* Vista Magazine, 20-21. www.vista-magonline.com

Dauncey, G. July 2006. *Winning the Cancer Game.* Common Ground, p. 24. http://www.common-ground.ca/iss/0607180/cg180_guy.shtml

Atkinson, L. 10:01am 4th July 2006. *You're eating the WRONG fruit and veg!* Daily Mail. http://www.dailymail.co.uk/pages/live/articles/health/dietfitness.html?in_article_id=393956&in_page_id=1798&in_a_source=

Herriot, C. Summer 2006. *The Missing Link.* GardenWise, British Columbia's Gardening Magazine, p. 12.

Schaefer, B., Burke, D. May/June 2006. *Natural Clues to Cancer Intervention.* Vista Magazine, 52-53. www.vistamagonline.com

Schaefer, B. Spring 2006. *Latest Developments in Salvestrol Therapy.* Health Action Magazine, 26-27.

Daniels, A. April 2006. *Salvestrols vs Cancer: The Story Continues.* Public Lecture held in Burnaby, B.C. DVD available from Health Action Network Society. http://www.hans.org/store/Cancer_Prevention

Burke, D. March 2006. *Latest Developments in Salvestrol Therapy.* Public Lecture held in Burnaby, B.C. DVD available from Health Action Network Society. http://www.hans.org/store/Cancer_Prevention

Dauncey, G. March 2006. *Organic Food And Cancer.* EcoNews http://www.earthfuture.com/econews/

Herriot, C. March 2006. *The Holy Grail For Cancer.* The Garden Path, www.earthfuture.com/gardenpath

Shannon, K. March 2006. *My Story: From Terminal Cancer to Long Life by Using Salvestrols.*

Schaefer, B. Winter 2006. *Breakthroughs In The Quest To Prevent and Cure Cancer: Professor Potter's BC Lecture Tour.* Health Action Magazine, 28-29.

Burke, D. Winter 2006. *Polymorphisms. What Are They And Why Are They Important?* Health Action Magazine, 26-27, 34.

Kuprowsky, S. Jan/Feb 2006. *Potential Cancer Breakthrough: The New-Found Cancer Killer Inside*

Certain Vegetables. Vista Magazine, 20-21. www.vistamagonline.com

Dauncey, G. Jan/Feb 2006. *Cancer, Fruit and Organic Farming: What Are We Doing Wrong?* Vista Magazine, 64-65. www.vistamagonline.com

Schaefer, B. Jan/Feb 2006. *Breakthroughs In The Quest To Cure Cancer.* The Herbal Collective, 29, 31. http://www.herbalcollective.ca

Frketich, K. Winter 2005/2006. *Cancer Research: Lecture Review.* British Columbia Naturopathic Association Bulletin, 12.

Thurnell-Read, J., M.Sc., KFRP. November 2005. *More On Salvestrols, Skin and Tumours.* Life-Work Potential.

Burke, D. Autumn 2005. *Salvestrols – A Natural Defence Against Cancer?* Health Action Magazine, 16-17. http://www.hans.org/magazine/173/Salvestrols-A-Natural-Defence-Against

Thurnell-Read, J., M.Sc., KFRP. October 2005. *Eczema, Psoriasis, Parkinson's & Tumours.* Life-Work Potential.

Thurnell-Read, J., M.Sc., KFRP. October 2005. *Skin Problems.* Health and Goodness.

Greene, M. Oct 13th, 2005. *U.K. Doctor Claims*

Food Enzymes Can Cure Cancer. The Martlet, Volume 58, Issue 10. http://www.hans.org/ newsletters/2005-Fall.pdf

Potter, G. September 2005. *Breakthroughs In The Quest To Prevent and Cure Cancer*. Public Lecture held in Vancouver, B.C. DVD available from Health Action Network Society. http://www. hans.org/store/Cancer_Prevention

Helen Knowles. 3 June, 2005. *Will Fruit and Vegetable Plant Salvestrols Save us from Cancers?* Herbsphere.   http://www.herbsphere.com/new_ page_10.htm

BNN: British Nursing News Online. Thursday, 27 January 2005 16:26. *Fruit and Veg Cure for Cancer.*   http://www.bnn-online.co.uk/news_ search.asp?TextChoice=salvestrol&TextChoice2= &Operator=AND&Year=2005

BBC News UK Edition, Thursday, 27 January, 2005, 11:45 GMT, *Fruit 'Could Provide Cancer Hope'.*   http://news.bbc.co.uk/1/hi/england/ leicestershire/4211223.stm

The Observer, Sunday January 2, 2005, *Fight Cancer With Food*. http://observer.guardian. co.uk/magazine/story/0,11913,1380969,00.html

Leicester Mercury, September 13, 2003. *Hope in his hands*. P. 11.

Kathryn Senior, (2002). *Molecular Explanation For Cancer-Preventive Properties Of Red Wine.* The Lancet Oncology, Vol. 3, No. 4, 01.

Cancer Research UK, Press Release, Tuesday 26 February 2002. *How A Plant's Anti-Fungal Defence May Protect Against Cancer* http://info.cancerresearchuk.org/pressoffice/pressreleases/2002/february/40684

BBC News Health, Tuesday, 26 February, 2002, 18:11 GMT, *Natural Defence Against Cancer.* http://news.bbc.co.uk/1/hi/health/1841709.stm

Britten, N., & Derbyshire, D. July, 2001. *Tumour-Destroying Drug 'May Be Cure For Cancer'* The Daily Telegraph, 28.

BBC News Health, Friday, 27 July, 2001, 17:09 GMT 18:09 UK, *Cancer Drug Raises Hopes Of Cure.* http://news.bbc.co.uk/1/hi/health/1460757.stm

RESEARCH REFERENCES

Attard G, Belldegrun AS, de Bono JS (2005). Selective blockade of androgenic steroid synthesis by novel lyase inhibitors as a therapeutic strategy for treating metastatic prostate cancer. *BJU Int.* **96** (9): 1241–6.

Attard G, Reid AHM, Yap TA, Raynaud F, Dowsett M, Settatree S, Barrett M, Parker C, Martins V, Folkerd E, Clark J, Cooper CS, Kaye SB, Dearnaley D, Lee G, de Bono JS (2008). Phase I Clinical Trial of a Selective Inhibitor of CYP17, Abiraterone Acetate, Confirms That Castration-Resistant Prostate Cancer Commonly Remains Hormone Driven. *Journal of Clinical Oncology* **26**: 4563.

Attard G, Reid A, A'Hern R, Parker C, Oommen N, Folkerd E, Messiou C, Molife L, Maier G, Thompson E, Olmos D, Sinha R, Lee G, Dowsett M, Kaye S, Dearnaley D, Kheoh T, Molina A, and de Bono J (2009). Selective Inhibition of CYP17 With Abiraterone Acetate Is Highly Active in the Treatment of Castration-Resistant Prostate Cancer. *Journal of Clinical Oncology*, **27**(23):3742-8.

Barnett JA, Urbauer DL, Murray GI, *et al.* (2007). Cytochrome P450 1B1 expression in glial cell tumors: an immunotherapeutic target. *Clin Cancer Res.* **13**: 3559-3567.

Bertz RJ, Granneman GR. (1997) Use of in vitro and in vivo data to estimate the likelihood of metabolic pharmacokinetic interactions. *Clin Pharmacokinet,* **32**: 210-58.

Burke, MD. (2009). The silent growth of cancer and its implications for nutritional protection. *British Naturopathic Journal,* **26**:1, 15-18.

Burke, MD, & Potter, G (2006). Salvestrols ... Natural Plant and Cancer Agents? *British Naturopathic Journal,* **23**:1,10-13.

Carnell D, Smith R, Daley F, et al. (2004). Target validation of cytochrome P450 CYP1B1 in prostate carcinoma with protein expression in associated hyperplastic and premalignant tissue. Int *J Radiat Oncol Biol Phys.* **58**: 500-509.

Chang JT, Chang H, Chen P, et al, (2007). Requirement of aryl hydrocarbon receptor overexpression for CYP1B1 up-regulation and cell growth in human lung adenocarcinomas. *Clin Cancer Res.* **13**: 38-45.

Chang H, Su J, Huang CC, *et al.* (2005). Using a combination of cytochrome P450 1B1 and b-catenin for early diagnosis and prevention of colorectal cancer. *Cancer Detect Prevent*. **29**: 562–569.

Dhaini HR, Thomas DG, Giordano TJ, Johnson TD, Biermann JS, Leu K, Hollenberg PF, Baker LH (2003). Cytochrome P450 CYP3A4/5 Expression as a Biomarker of Outcome in Osteosarcoma. *Journal of Clinical Oncology*, **21**: 2481-2485.

Dorai T, Aggarwall BB (2004) Role of chemoprotective agents in cancer therapy. *Cancer Letters* **215**: 129-140.

Downie D, McFadyen M, Rooney P, et al. (2005). Profiling cytochrome P450 expression in ovarian cancer:identification of prognostic markers. *Clin Cancer Res*. **11**: 7369-7375.

Everett S, McErlane VM, McLeod K, et al. (2007). Profiling cytochrome P450 CYP1 enzyme expression in primary melanoma and disseminated disease utilizing spectral imaging microscopy (SIM). *J Clin Oncology*. **25**: 8556.

Ferrigni, NR, McLaughlin JL (1984). Use of potato disc and brine shrimp bioassays to detect activity and isolate piceatannol as the antileukemic principle from the seeds of *Euphorbia lagascae*. *J. Nat. Prod*. **47**:347-352.

Fuller F (April 26th, 2011). An Orthomolecular Approach to Cancer. *4th Annual Cancer*

Prevention and Healing Event, Health Action Network Society, Burnaby, B.C., Canada.

Gibson, P. et al., (2003) Cytochrome P450 1B1 (CYP1B1) Is Overexpressed in Human Colon Adenocarcinomas Relative to Normal Colon: Implications for Drug Development. *Molecular Cancer Therapeutics*, **2**: 527-534.

Greer ML, Richman PI, Barber PR, et al, (2004). Cytochrome P450 1B1 (CYP1B1) is expressed during the malignant progression of head and neck squamous cell carcinoma (HNSCC). *Proc Amer Cancer Res*. **45**: Abstract #3701.

Gribben, J.G. et al., (2005) Unexpected association between induction of immunity to the universal tumor antigen CYP1B1 and response to next therapy. *Clinical Cancer Research*, **11**: 4430-4436.

Haas S, Pierl C, Harth V, *et al*. (2006). Expression of xenobiotic and steroid hormone metabolizing enzymes in human breast carcinomas. *Int J Cancer*. **119**: 1785-1791.

Hanna IH, Dawling S, Roodi N, F. Peter Guengerich FP, Parl FF, (2000). Cytochrome P450 *1B1 (CYP1B1)* Pharmacogenetics: Association of Polymorphisms with Functional Differences in Estrogen Hydroxylation Activity. *Cancer Research* **60**: 3440-3444.

Hayes CL, Spink DC, Spink BC, Cao JQ, Walker NJ, and Thomas R. Sutter TR (1996) 17-Estradiol hydroxylation catalyzed by human cytochrome P450 1B1. *Medical Sciences,* **93**: 9776-9781.

Hsieh TC, Wu JM (1999) Differential effects on growth, cell cycle arrest, and induction of apoptosis by resveratrol in human prostate cancer cell lines. *Experimental Cell Research* 249(1): 109-15.

Jang M, Cai L, Udeani G, Slowing K, Thomas C, Beecher C, Fong H, Farnsworth N, Kinghorn A, Mehta R, Moon R, Pezzuto J, (1997) Cancer Chemopreventive Activity of Resveratrol, a Natural Product Derived from Grapes. *Science* **275**: 218 – 220.

Jang M, Pezzuto J, (1999) Cancer Chemopreventive Activity of Resveratrol. *Drugs Exp Clin Res* **25**: 65-77.

Kim JH, Stansbury KH, Walker NJ, Trush MA, Strickland PT, Sutter TR (1998) Metabolism of benzo[a]pyrene and benzo[a]pyrene-7, 8-diol by human cytochrome P450 1B1. *Carcenogenesis* **19**: 1847-1853.

Kumarakulasingham M, Rooney PH, Dundas SR, *et al.* (2005). Cytochrome P450 profile of colorectal cancer: identification of markers of prognosis. *Clin Cancer Res.* **11**: 3758-3765.

Lin P, Chang H, Ho WL, *et al.* (2003). Association of aryl hydrocarbon receptor and cytochrome

P4501B1 expressions in human non-small cell lung cancers. *Lung Cancer.* **42**: 255-261.

Li DN, Seidel A, Pritchard MP, Wolf CR, Friedberg T. (2000). Polymorphisms in P450 CYP1B1 affect the conversion of estradiol to the potentially carcinogenic metabolite 4-hydroxyestradiol. *Pharmacogenetics.* **10** : 343-53.

Li NC, & Wakeman M. (October 2009) High-performance liquid chromatography comparison of eight beneficial secondary plant metabolites in the flesh and peel or 15 varieties of apples. *The Pharmaceutical Journal*, supplement Vol. **283**, B40.

Li NC, & Wakeman M. (2009) High-performance liquid chromatography comparison of eight beneficial secondary plant metabolites in the flesh and peel or 15 varieties of apples. *Journal of Pharmacy and Pharmacology*, supplement **1**, A132.

Maecker B, Sherr DH, Vonderheide RH, von Bergwelt-Baildon MS, Hirano N, Anderson KS, Xia Z, Butler MO, Wucherpfennig KW, O'Hara C, Cole G, Kwak SS, Ramstedt U, Tomlinson AJ, Chicz RM, Nadler LM, and Schultze JL. (2003) The shared tumor-associated antigen cytochrome P450 1B1 is recognized by specific cytotoxic T cells. *Blood.* Nov 1;102(9):3287-94.

Magee, J.B., Smith, B.J., and Rimando, A. (2002). Resveratrol Content of Muscadine Berries is Affected by Disease Control Spray Program.

Journal of the American Society for Horticultural Science, **37**:358-361.

McFadyen MCE, Melvin WT, Murray GI (2004) Cytochrome *P*450 enzymes: Novel options for cancer therapeutics. *Molecular Cancer Therapeutics*, **3**: 363-371.

McFadyen MCE, Melvin WT, Murray GI (2004) Cytochrome *P*450 CYP1B1 activity in renal cell carcinoma. *British Journal of Cancer* **91**: 966-971.

McFadyen MCE, Cruickshank ME, Miller ID, et al. (2001) Cytochrome *P*450 CYP1B1 overexpression in primary and metastatic ovarian cancer. *British Journal of Cancer* **85**:242–6.

McFadyen MCE, Breeman S, Payne S, et al. Immunohistochemical localization of cytochrome *P*450 CYP1B1 in breast cancer with monoclonal antibodies specific for CYP1B1. *Journal of Histochemistry and Cytochemistry,* 1999; **47**:1457–64.

McKay J, Melvin W, Ahsee A, Ewen S, Greenlee W, Marcus C, Burke M, Murray G (1995) Expression Of Cytochrome-P450 Cyp1b1 In Breast-Cancer *FEBS Letters* **374**(2): 270-272.

Michael M, Doherty MM. (2005) Tumoral Drug Metabolism: Overview and Its Implications for Cancer Therapy. *Journal of Clinical Oncology,* **23,** 205-229.

Murray GI, Melvin WT, Greenlee WF, Burke MD, (2001) Regulation, function, and tissue-specific expression of cytochrome P450 CYP1B1. *Annual Review of Pharmacology and Toxicology.* **41**: 297-316.

Murray GI, Taylor MC, McFadyen MCE, McKay JA, Greenlee WF, Burke MD, Melvin WT (1997) Tumor specific expression of cytochrome P450 CYP 1B1. *Cancer Research,* **57**: 3026-3031.

Murray GI, McKay JA, Weaver RJ, et al, (1993) Cytochrome P450 expression is a common molecular event in soft tissue sarcomas. *Journal of Pathology,* **171**:49–52,

Oyama, T, Morita, M, Isse, T, et al, (2005). Immunohistochemical evaluation of cytochrome P450 (CYP) and P53 in breast cancer. *Front Biosci.* **10**: 1156-1161.

Patterson LH, Murray GI (2002). Tumour cytochrome P450 and drug activation. *Current Pharmaceutical Design,* **8**:1335-1347.

Port J, Yamaguchi K, Du B, De Lorenzo M, Chang M, Heerdt P, Kopelovich L, Marcus C, Altorki N, Subbaramaiah K, Dannenberg A (2004). Tobacco smoke induces CYP1B1 in the aerodigestive tract. Carcinogenesis, **25**(11): 2275-2281.

Potter GA, Burke DM (2006) Salvestrols – Natural Products with Tumour Selective Activity. *Journal of Orthomolecular Medicine,* 21, **1**: 34-36.

Potter GA (2002) <u>The role of CYP 1B1 as a tumour suppressor enzyme</u>. *British Journal of Cancer,* **86** (Suppl 1), S12, 2002.

Potter GA, Patterson LH, Wanogho E et al (2002) <u>The cancer preventative agent resveratrol is converted to the anticancer agent piceatonnal by the cytochrome P450 enzyme CYP 1B1</u>. *British Journal of Cancer,* **86**: 774-778.

Potter GA, Patterson LH, Burke MD (2001) <u>Aromatic hydroxylation activated (AHA) prodrugs</u>. *US Patent 6,214,886.*

Prud'homme A, (2009) <u>Comparative Analysis of Polyphenolic Residues from Grape Pomace to Contain Wine</u>. *Training report, Département Chimie, Université du Maine.*

<u>Report Of The Independent Vitamin Safety Review Panel</u>. (May 23, 2006). *Orthomolecular Medicine News Service.*

Rochat B, Morsman JM, Murray GI, Figg WD, McLeod HL. (2001) <u>Human CYP1B1 and Anticancer Agent Metabolism: Mechanism for Tumor-Specific Drug Inactivation?</u> *Pharmacology and Experimental Therapeutics* **296**, 537-541.

Rodriguez-Melendez R, Griffin JB & Zempleni J (2004) <u>Biotin Supplementation Increases Expression of the Cytochrome P_{450} 1B1 Gene in Jurkat Cells, Increasing the Occurrence of Single-</u>

Stranded DNA Breaks. *The Journal of Nutrition*, **134**:2222-2228.

Schaefer BA, Dooner C, Burke DM, Potter GA, (2010) Nutrition and Cancer: Further Case Studies Involving Salvestrol. *Journal of Orthomolecular Medicine*, **25**, 1: 17-23.

Schaefer, B.A. (April 2010) Early Cancer Detection. Proceedings of the *39th Orthomolecular Medicine Today Conference, Vancouver, B.C.*

Schaefer BA, Hoon LT, Burke DM, Potter GA, (2007) Nutrition and Cancer: Salvestrol Case Studies. *Journal of Orthomolecular Medicine*, **22**, 4: 1-6.

Shimada T, Hayes CL, Yamazaki H, Amin S, Hecht SS, Guengerich FP, Sutter TR (1996) Activation of chemically diverse procarcinogens by human cytochrome P450 1B1. *Cancer Research* **56**: 2979-2984.

Skov T, Lynge E, Maarup B, Olsen J, Rørth M, Winthereik H [1990]. Risk for physicians handling antineoplastic drugs [letter to the editor]. *The Lancet* **336**:1446.

Skov T, Maarup B, Olsen J, Rørth M, Winthereik H, Lynge E [1992]. Leukaemia and reproductive outcome among nurses handling antineoplastic drugs. *Br J Ind Med* **49**:855–861.

Sorsa M, Hemminki K, et al. (1985). Occupational exposure to anticancer drugs--potential and real hazards. *Mutation Research* **154**:135-149.

Stellman JM, Zoloth, SR (1986) Cancer chemotherapeutic agents as occupational hazards: A literature review. *Cancer Investigation* **4**:2, 127-135.

Su, J, Lin, P, Wang, C, et al, (2009). Overexpression of cytochrome P450 1B1 in advanced non-small cell lung cancer: a potential therapeutic target. *Anticancer Res.* **29**: 509-515.

Surh YJ, Hurh YJ, Kang JY (1999) Resveratrol, an antioxidant in red wine, induces apoptosis in human promyelocytic leukemia (HL-60) cells. *Cancer Letters,* June 1: **140**(1-2): 1-10.

Tan, H. August/September (2007). Can Food Really be Your Medicine? *Townsend Letter*, 116-119.

Tan HL, K. Beresford K, Butler PC, Potter GA, & Burke MD, (2007). Salvestrols – Natural Anticancer Prodrugs in The Diet. *J. Pharm. Pharmacol.* **59**: S158

Tan, HL, Butler PC, Burke MD, & Potter GA, (2007). Salvestrols: A New Perspective in Nutritional Research.*Journal of Orthomolecular Medicine*, 2007; **22**(1): 39-47.

Tokizane, T. et al., (2005) Cytochrome P450

CYP1B1 is overexpressed and regulated by hypo-methylation in prostate cancer. *Clinical Cancer Research*, **11**: 5793-5801.

Ware WR, (2009) Nutrition and the Prevention and Treatment of Cancer: Association of Cytochrome P450 CYP1B1 With the Role of Fruit and Fruit Extracts. *Integrative Cancer Therapies*, **8**, 1: 22-28.

Ware WR, (2009) P450 CYP1B1 mediated fluo-rescent tumor markers: A potentially useful ap-proach for photodynamic therapy, diagnosis and establishing surgical margins. *Medical Hypotheses*, **72**: 67-70.

Zhao Z, Kosinska W, Khmelnitsky M, Cavalieri EL, Rogan EG, Chakravarti D, Sacks PG, Guttenplan JB, (2006). Mutagenic activity of 4-hydroxyestradiol, but not 2-hydroxyestradiol, in BB rat2 embryonic cells, and the mutational spec-trum of 4-hydroxyestradiol. *Chemical Research in Toxicology*, **19**: 475-479.

FOR MORE INFORMATION:

Health Action Network Society#202 — 5262 Rumble Street Burnaby, B.C., V5J 2B6 CANADA www.hans.org

International Society for Orthomolecular Medicine 16 Florence Avenue Toronto Ontario M2N 1E9 CANADA www.orthomed.org

Canadian Association of Holistic Nutrition Professionals CAHN-Pro 150 Consumers Road Toronto, Ontario M2J 1P9 www.cahnpro.org

APPENDIX 1.

EVIDENCE OF CYP1B1 EXPRESSION IN CANCER CELLS.

CANCER:	REFERENCE:
acute lymphocytic leukaemia	Maecker B, et al, 2003
acute myeloid leukaemia	Maecker B, et al, 2003 Michael M, Doherty MM. 2005
bladder cancer	Carnell, D, et al, 2004 Murray GI, et al, 1997 Patterson LH, Murray GI, 2002
brain cancer	Barnett, JA, et al, 2007 Murray GI, et al, 1997
breast cancer	Haas S, et al, 2006 McFadyen MCE, et al, 1999 Murray GI, et al, 1997 Maecker B, et al, 2003 Michael M, Doherty MM. 2005 Oyama T, et al, 2005 Patterson LH, Murray GI, 2002

colon/colorectal cancer	Chang H, et al, 2005
	Kumarakulasingham M, et al, 2005
	Murray GI, et al, 1997
	Maecker B, et al, 2003
	Michael M, Doherty MM. 2005
connective tissue	Murray GI, et al, 1997
head and neck	Greer, ML, et al, 2004
kidney cancer (renal cell carcinoma)	McFadyen MCE, et al, 2004
	Michael M, Doherty MM. 2005
	Murray GI, et al, 1997
lung cancer	Chang, JT, et al 2007
	Lin P, et al, 2003
	Murray GI, et al, 1997
	Maecker B, et al, 2003
	Michael M, Doherty MM. 2005
	Patterson LH, Murray GI, 2002
	Su J, et al, 2009
liver cancer	Patterson LH, Murray GI, 2002
lymph nodes	Murray GI, et al, 1997
lymphoma	Maecker B, et al, 2003
melanoma	Maecker B, et al, 2003
multiple myeloma	Maecker B, et al, 2003
non-Hodgin's lymphoma	Murray GI, et al, 1997
	Michael M, Doherty MM. 2005
oesophageal cancer	Murray GI, et al, 1997
	Maecker B, et al, 2003
	Michael M, Doherty MM. 2005
osteosarcoma	Dhaini HR, et al, 2003

ovarian carcinoma	Downie D, et al, 2005 Murray GI, et al, 1997 Maecker B, et al, 2003 McFadyen MCE, et al, 2001 Michael M, Doherty MM. 2005
prostate cancer	Carnell, D, et al, 2004 Patterson LH, Murray GI, 2002 Michael M, Doherty MM. 2005
rhabdomyosarcoma	Maecker B, et al, 2003
skin cancer	Everett, SVM, et al, 2007 Murray GI, et al, 1997
soft tissue sarcomas	Michael M, Doherty MM. 2005 Murray GI, et al, 1993
stomach cancer	Murray GI, et al, 1997 Michael M, Doherty MM. 2005
testicular cancer	Murray GI, et al, 1997 Michael M, Doherty MM. 2005
uterine cancer	Murray GI, et al, 1997 Michael M, Doherty MM. 2005
etc.	

Note that many cancers other than those listed above express CYP1B1. This list simply highlights the diversity of cancers that express this enzyme. The list was derived from studies that were specifically testing various cancers for the presence of CYP1B1.

APPENDIX 2.

DIET AND CANCER. WHAT HEALTH DEPARTMENTS AND ORGANISATIONS ARE SAYING

"… about 40 per cent of men and 35 per cent of women will develop cancer during their lifetime just over 25 per cent of men and 20 per cent of women will die of cancer."

Health Canada. *Cancer: What's your risk?* http://www.hc-sc.gc.ca/english/feature/magazine/ 2001_04/cancer.htm

"Current evidence suggests that diet-related factors account for about 30% of all cancers in developed countries."

Public Health Agency of Canada. *Progress Report on Cancer Control in Canada. Cancer Prevention. Diet.* http://www.phac-aspc.gc.ca/ publicat/prccc-relccc/chap_3_e.htm

"Fruit and vegetable consumption is protective for a variety of cancers"

Public Health Agency of Canada. Centre for Chronic Disease Prevention and Control http://www.phac-aspc.gc.ca/ccdpc-cpcmc/ cancer/index_e.html

"Cancer with convincing or probable evidence for prevention by vegetable and fruit consumption …: Mouth, Throat, Esophagus, Stomach, Colon, Rectum, Pancreas, Larynx, Lung, Bladder"

Cancer Care Ontario. *Media Release*

"Evidence indicates that a diet high in fruits and vegetables reduces the risk of several types of cancer, particularly cancers of the gastrointestinal tract (mouth, pharynx, esophagus, stomach, colon and rectum)."

Public Health Agency of Canada. *Progress Report on Cancer Control in Canada. Cancer Prevention: Diet* http://www.phac-aspc.gc.ca/publicat/prccc-relccc/chap_3_e.html

"Why focus on vegetables and fruit for cancer prevention? Vegetables and fruit are good for us for many reasons, but the strongest evidence for promoting a diet high in produce relates to the risk of cancer. The American Institute for Cancer Research and the World Cancer Research Fund commissioned a review of research from around the world in 1997. The research review concluded that 'consumption of five servings or more of a variety of vegetables and fruit could, by itself, decrease overall cancer incidence by at least 20%.'"

Alberta Cancer Board. *Cancer Prevention. Simply Healthy Campaign: Campaign Rationale* http://www.cancerboard.ab.ca/cancer/simply-healthy/campaign.html

FACTS:

Up to 2.7 million lives could be saved annually with sufficient fruit and vegetable consumption. Low fruit and vegetable intake is among the top 10 selected risk factors for global mortality. Worldwide, low intake of fruits and vegetables is estimated to cause about 19% of gastrointestinal cancer, about 31% of ischaemic heart disease and 11% of stroke."

> **World Health Organization**. *Global Strategy on Diet, Physical Activity and Health. Fruit, vegetables and NCD prevention.* http://www. who.int/dietphysicalactivity/publications/ facts/fruit/en/

"A high-level international review on fruit and vegetable consumption and cancer risk, coordinated by the International Agency for Research on Cancer (IARC), concluded that eating fruits and vegetables may lower the risk of cancer, particularly cancers of the gastrointestinal tract. IARC estimates that the preventable fraction of cancer due to low fruit and vegetable intake falls into the range of 5-12 % and up to 20-30% for upper gastro-intestinal tract cancers world-wide."

> **World Health Organization**. *Global Strategy on Diet, Physical Activity and Health. Fruit, vegetables and NCD prevention.* http://www. who.int/dietphysicalactivity/publications/ facts/fruit/en/

Cancer accounts for 7.1 million deaths annually (12.5% of the global total).

Dietary factors account for about 30% of all cancers in Western Countries and approximately up to 20% in developing countries; diet is second only to tobacco as a preventable cause. Approximately 20 million people suffer from cancer; a figure projected to rise to 30 million within 20 years.

The number of new cases annually is estimated to rise from 10 million to 15 million by 2020.

More than half of all cancer cases occur in developing countries."

> **World Health Organization.** *Global Strategy on Diet, Physical Activity and Health. Cancer: diet and physical activity's impact.* http://www. who.int/dietphysicalactivity/publications/ facts/cancer/en/

APPENDIX 3.

THE GREEN AND RED DIET

As this research found its way into the popular press Professor Potter's Cancer Drug Discovery Group started to receive requests for help from people suffering from cancer. The first response was to embody the knowledge that they had gained into a dietary recommendation. This became known as the "Green and Red Diet".

Professor Potter's dietary recommendations follow:

"Primarily have a vegetarian diet including fruits, vegetables, and herbs. Following this advice, and being selective about both the type and quality of produce you consume will help to maximise your dietary intake of the important salvestrols. Wherever possible eat organic.

This is the easily remembered 'Green and Red' diet, where the savoury course includes the green vegetables and herbs, and the dessert course includes the red fruits. It is no accident that as a species we prefer to eat savoury foods first and sweet foods after. This preference has evolved, we believe, to maximise the absorption and activation of vital nutrients, such as salvestrols.

For the savoury course the vegetables should be cooked as lightly as possible, and the goodness retained in the food. For example, if vegetables are boiled use the water to make gravy or sauces. Roasting whole vegetables is also a good way of retaining the plants goodness.

The fruits and vegetables with the highest salvestrol contents are listed below:"

FRUITS:		
All Red		**Other**
blackberries	loganberries	apples
blackcurrants	mulberries	dates
blueberries	plums	figs
cranberries	raspberries	mangoes
damsons	redcurrants	pears
grapes	strawberries	pineapples
		tangerines

VEGETABLES:		
All Green		
asparagus	lettuces	cucumbers
broad beans	savoy	gherkins
broccoli	spinach	gourds
brussels sprouts	watercress	marrows
cabbages	**Other**	melons
chard	artichokes (globe)	peppers (all colours)
Chinese leaf	avocado	pumpkins

garden peas	bean sprouts	salad rocket (arugula)
green beans	calabrese	squashes
kales	cauliflower	wild carrots
kohlrabi	celery	zucchini

HERBS:		
Common herbs	**Medicinal herbs**	
basil	burdock	plantain
mint	chamomile	rooibosh
parsley	dandelion	rose hip
rosemary	hawthorn	skullcap
sage	lemon verbena	
thyme	milk thistle root	

THE MAIN SALVESTROL RICH PLANT FAMILIES:

COMPOSITAE FAMILY INCLUDES:	
globe artichoke	dandelion
thistle	burdock
milk thistle	chamomile

ROSACEA FAMILY INCLUDES:	
rose hip	hawthorn

BRASSICA FAMILY INCLUDES:	
cabbage	
broccoli	spring cabbage
cauliflower	savoy cabbage

The Green and Red Diet is reproduced here with the kind permission of Professor Gerry Potter.

APPENDIX 4.

SAMPLE SALVESTROL RICH RECIPES

Artichokes in Dipping Sauce

INGREDIENTS:

4 medium artichokes;	1 chopped onion;
2 cloves garlic (minced);	2 Tbls. minced fresh mint;
½ tsp. crumbled rosemary;	¼ cup olive oil (stone ground);
2 Tbls. lemon juice;	½ cup cider vinegar;
½ cup water;	½ tsp. sea salt.

Rinse artichokes and cut 1 inch off the tops. With scissors, trim off the thorny tips of the remaining leaves. In a large saucepan, sauté the onion, garlic, mint and rosemary in oil. Add lemon juice, vinegar, water and sea salt. Place artichokes in seasoned broth; cover and simmer until tender, about 40 minutes. Allow to cool in the broth. To serve, place each artichoke in a bowl with some of the broth to use as a dipping sauce.

SALVESTROL POINTS PER SERVING 5 (20 POINTS IF ORGANIC PRODUCE USED)

Avocado Ahdi

INGREDIENTS:

2 small avocados;

½ cup chopped red bell pepper;

¼ cup chopped green bell pepper;

¼ cup diced wild carrots;

¼ cup chopped cucumber;

¼ cup chopped tomatoes;

¼ chopped red onions;

10 Spanish olives - chopped;

juice of 1 lime; ½ tsp.

sea salt; pepper to taste;

Tabasco to taste;

chopped fresh coriander.

Cut the avocados in half lengthways very carefully, discard the pits and carefully scoop out the shells. Reserve the shells; Chop the flesh finely and set aside. Combine the chopped vegetables and olives. Season with the lime juice, sea salt, pepper and Tabasco. Add the avocado and toss lightly. Take care not to break up the avocado too much. Gently mound the salad into the avocado shells or on a bed of fresh spinach leaves. Garnish lightly with coriander.

SALVESTROL POINTS PER SERVING 6 (24 POINTS IF ORGANIC PRODUCE USED)

Fresh Asparagus in Butter Sauce

INGREDIENTS (serves 4 persons):

2 dozen fresh, thin asparagus;

1 cup of butter;

2 fresh cloves of garlic;

2 tsp. lemon juice;

1 tsp. of parsley flakes;

½ tsp. of grated lemon rind;

parsley sprigs.

Wash spears and snap off white ends, cut spears into bias-sliced chucks about 2" long. In a wok or frying pan, melt butter. Press garlic through a press and add with lemon juice and parsley flakes to butter. Heat contents over medium-high heat. Add asparagus and stir constantly until vegetables are crisp-tender. Remove asparagus to warm serving dish. Add lemon rind to butter sauce in pan. Heat until bubbly and pour over asparagus. Garnish with parsley sprigs and serve immediately.

SALVESTROL POINTS PER SERVING 5 (20 POINTS IF ORGANIC PRODUCE USED)

Artichoke and Tomato Chicken

INGREDIENTS (serves 6 persons):

28-oz. of whole tomatoes;	½ tsp. sea salt;
9-oz. artichoke heart;	¼ tsp. ground pepper;
½ cup of dry white wine;	6 chicken legs;
½ cup of reserved tomato juice;	2 tsp. lemon zest, grated;
1 tsp. dried tarragon;	2 Tbls. parsley, chopped.

Drain the tomatoes and reserve ½ cup of juice. Slit open the tomatoes and pick out the seeds, drain the juices and finely chop the flesh. Combine the tomatoes with the artichoke hearts in a large skillet and place over moderate heat. Add the wine and reserved tomatoes juice and bring to a boil. Stir in the tarragon, sea salt and pepper. Arrange the chicken legs in a single layer on top of the tomatoes and artichokes. Cover and simmer for about 25 minutes, or until the chickens is no longer pink at the bone when slashed. Stir in the lemon zest. Arrange the chicken on a platter, spoon the sauce over and sprinkle with the parsley.

SALVESTROL POINTS PER SERVING 6 (24 POINTS IF ORGANIC PRODUCE USED)

INDEX

gastrointestinal 128, 129
genes 11
genome 1
George Bernard Shaw 10
Gerry Potter viii, ix, 5, 6, 7, 8, 17, 18, 19, 20, 21, 22, 23, 24, 25, 26, 28, 32, 35, 39, 49, 50, 51, 52, 68, 72, 80, 95, 96, 97, 102, 103, 104, 107, 109, 112, 118, 119, 120, 121, 131, 134
gherkins 132
glaucoma 47
glycoside 87, 88, 90, 97, 98
gourds 132
Graham Boyes ix
grape 23, 43, 44, 45, 58, 100, 132
Green and Red Diet ix, 50, 131, 134, 135
guava 59

H

halibut 58
Harry Foster 94
hawthorn 133, 134
Health Action Magazine 47, 103, 104, 105, 106, 107, 108
Health Action Network Society ix, 104, 107, 109, 114, 123
Helen Bailey ix
Henry Ford 77
herb 28, 39, 51, 61, 66
Herbal Apothecary 50, 51
herbalism 27

herbicide 40
Hippocrates 28
hplc 88, 89, 98
hydrophilic 27, 72, 101
hydroxylation 11, 19, 24, 115, 119

I

Ian Morrison ix
immunohistochemical 13
inhibitor 6, 16, 18, 46, 97
inhibitors 15, 39, 46, 52, 96, 111
Institute of Cancer Research 6
International Agency for Research on Cancer 129
Iraida Garcia ix
iron 11, 57, 58, 59, 60, 61
Isabelle Eini ix
ischaemic heart disease 129

J

Jim Stott ix

K

kale 57, 133
kales 133
Kathy Thammavong ix
Katolen Yardley ix
Kevin Coyne ix
kidney 2, 88, 125
kiwifruit 59
kohlrabi 133

U

V

W

Z

THE AUTHOR

The author was educated in Victoria, B.C., Canada and Oxford, England, obtained a B.Sc., and M.Sc., degree from the University of Victoria and a Doctor of Philosophy (D.Phil.) degree from Oxford University in England (Wolfson College). After these studies were completed he chose to return to Canada. After two years as a research fellow in Ottawa he returned to Victoria where he currently lives with his wife and his two children. A fondness for England continues and he returns to England on a regular basis. He has published and lectured on a broad array of topics including psychometrics, pattern recognition, visual perception, knowledge acquisition, artificial intelligence, laboratory medicine and cancer research. The author serves on the Board of Directors of companies in Canada and England.